Secondary Traumatic Stress: Treatment and Management

MARIO VAN TONDER

Secondary Traumatic Stress: Treatment and Management

A study into the efficacy of the action centred personological treatment plan for emergency rescue workers

VDM Verlag Dr. Müller

Imprint

Bibliographic information by the German National Library: The German National Library lists this publication at the German National Bibliography; detailed bibliographic information is available on the Internet at http://dnb.d-nb.de.

Cover image: www.purestockx.com

Publisher:
VDM Verlag Dr. Müller Aktiengesellschaft & Co. KG , Dudweiler Landstr. 125 a, 66123 Saarbrücken, Germany,
Phone +49 681 9100-698, Fax +49 681 9100-988,
Email: info@vdm-verlag.de

Zugl.: Johannesburg, University of Johannesburg, TU,Diss.,2006

Produced in USA and UK by:
Lightning Source Inc., La Vergne, Tennessee, USA
Lightning Source UK Ltd., Milton Keynes, UK
BookSurge LLC, 5341 Dorchester Road, Suite 16, North Charleston, SC 29418, USA

ISBN: 978-3-8364-5405-6

CHAPTER ONE

INTRODUCTION

1.1 Introduction:

Worldwide there has been an increased awareness of occupational safety. In the UK the Department of Health (1998) recently aimed to "ensure that people are protected from the harm to their health that certain jobs can cause" (p51). Sabin-Farrel and Turpin (2003) state that in the USA and other countries occupational health projects are viewed as being important both for staff wellbeing as well as productivity, and performance. In South Africa Employee Wellbeing Programmes/ Services are on the increase in the corporate sector, indicating managements' awareness and acknowledgement of work stress and it's impact on staff.

Various contributing factors to work stress in the health sector include: aspects of organizations, job role, demands and characteristics, workload, work environment, or personality traits. Some of these factors may combine to make work in the health/rescue services inherently stressful (Sabin-Farrel and Turpin, 2003).

A specific form of occupational stress became apparent in theory over the past two decades in health service staff. The effort and skill needed to help others in need may be very rewarding when rescue workers are successful in a particular project. But when efforts are met with failure or when they experience long periods of strain the rescue workers may, themselves experience suffering.

Charles Figley (1995) coined the phrase: "the cost to caring". He implies that it is not only organizational or workplace factors that contribute to stress and ill health in healthcare workers, but also the aspects of the type of work that they are required to do. This he calls this Compassion Fatigue/Secondary Traumatic Stress.

Soon after the recognition of traumatisation in the 1970's it became clear that helpers, themselves may be affected in a secondary way. The terminologies that have been used in literature to describe the phenomenon vary considerably (see below). Many definitions overlap, contradict or negate each other with limited or no theoretical foundation. The efforts seem to be in validifying rather than falsifying latter concepts.

Criticism on the validity of such construct suggests that if PTSD can be best conceptualised as socially constructed rather than a psychopathological (Summerfield, 2001) and that trauma debriefing programmes may be "medicalising" normal distress to trauma (Rose, Bisson and Wessley, 2002), how can we rightfully talk of secondary traumatic stress?

True to the field of traumatology there are numerous points of view which have to be considered in order to make the concepts operational.

1.2   Historical context:

Trauma can be viewed as one of the oldest conditions in human developmental history. Ironically, only in the past 140 years has it enjoyed any scientific recognition. During the United States Civil War (1861-1865) a condition described as "Soldier's Heart" was recorded.

This term was replaced by Jacob da Costa in 1871 with what he called "irritable Heart Syndrome".

During World War I the debate on the etiology of "psychoneuroses" was revived.
Theorists were divided as to whether symptoms of: paralysis, tremor, delirium,
amnesia etc. were caused by physical or psychical origins. Oppenheim extended
his peacetime theory of the basis of "traumatic neuroses/shell shock", such as
follow a railway accident, and which he believed to be caused by "physical
commotion of the nervous system". It was during this time that the PIE-model was
used based on three principles of intervention; close to the battle zone (proximity),
as soon as possible (immediacy), and with the expectation of returning to duty
(expectancy) (Bisson, 2003).

Similar terminologies such as: "combat neuroses" or "operational fatigue" were
used during World War II. General Marshall held structured group debriefings on
the battlefield as soon as possible after the action. One of the main functions of
these meetings was information gathering; however Marshall noted that the
emotional effects of the debriefings were morale building, ventilation of negative
feelings and generally a positive experience for the soldiers (Bisson, 2003).

From the former several trauma diagnostic terminologies developed. The following
diagnostic terminologies are relevant to this study.

1.3   Posttraumatic Stress Disorder: etiology, definition and description

First mention of the term Posttraumatic Stress Disorder was made during the
Vietnam War aftermath in the 1970's. However this did not end the longstanding
controversy in psychological practice about the cause of mental illness that follows
an extremely traumatic experience (Horowitz, 1986).

The uncertainty revolves around the issue of whether the severity of the
trauma or the pre-morbid psychological vulnerability of the person involved is the
most important factor. In both the DSM-I and DSM-II conceptualizations of trauma,
it was described as an acute, time-limited phenomena that diminished unless

some pre-existing character pathology was present which would contribute to symptom maintenance Green, Grace, Lindy, Gleser, and Leonard (1990).

In contrast to the former the DSM-III emphasized the central etiological role of traumatic events in its formulation of posttraumatic stress disorders (American Psychiatric Association, 1980). This change in classification followed in line with the former mentioned debate after the first and second world wars, which now continued in the aftermath of the Vietnam War.

In the DSM-IV Posttraumatic Stress Disorder has been described as follow (American Psychiatric Association, 1994: pp424-425):

"The essential feature of Posttraumatic stress Disorder is the development of characteristic symptoms following exposure to an extreme traumatic stressor involving direct personal experience of an event that involves actual or threatened death or serious injury, or other threat to one's physical integrity; or witnessing an event that involves death, injury, or a threat to the physical integrity of another person; or learning about unexpected or violent death, serious harm, or threat of death experienced by a family member or other close associate (Criterion A1). The person's response to the event must involve intense fear, helplessness, or horror (or in children the response must involve disorganized or agitated behavior) (Criterion A2). The characteristic symptoms resulting from the exposure to the extreme trauma include persistent re-experiencing of the traumatic event (Criterion B), persistent avoidance of stimuli associated with the trauma and numbing of general responsiveness (Criterion C), and persistent symptoms of increased arousal (Criterion D). The full symptom picture must be present for more than 1 month (Criterion E), and the disturbance must cause significant distress or impairment in social, occupational, or other important areas of functioning (Criterion F).

Traumatic events that are experienced directly include, but are not limited to, military combat, violent personal assault (sexual assault, physical attack, robbery, and mugging), being kidnapped, being taken hostage, terrorist attack, torture, incarceration as a prisoner of war or in a concentration camp, natural or manmade disasters, severe automobile accidents, or being diagnosed with a life-threatening illness. For children, sexually traumatic events may include developmentally inappropriate sexual experiences without threatened or actual violence or injury.

Witnessed events include, but are not limited to, observing the serious injury or unnatural death of another person due to violent assault, accident, war, or disaster or unexpectedly witnessing a dead body or body parts. Events experienced by others that are learned about include, but are not limited to, violent personal assault, serious accident, or serious injury experienced by a family member or a close friend; learning about the sudden, unexpected death of a family member a close friend; or learning that one's child has a life-threatening disease.

The disorder may be especially severe or long lasting when the stressor is of human design (e.g. torture, rape). The likelihood of developing this disorder may increase as the intensity of and physical proximity to the stressor increase.

The traumatic event can be re-experienced in various ways. Commonly the person has recurrent and intrusive recollections of the event (Criterion B1) or recurrent distressing dreams during which the event is replayed (Criterion B2). In rare instances, the person experienced dissociative states that last from a few seconds to several hours, or even days, during which components of the event are relived and the person behaves as though experiencing the event at that moment (Criterion B3).

Intense psychological distress (Criterion B4) or physiological reactivity (Criterion B5) often occurs when the person is exposed to triggering events that resemble or symbolize an aspect of the traumatic event (e.g. anniversaries of the traumatic event; cold, snowy weather or uniformed guards for survivors of death camps in cold climates; hot humid weather for combat veterans of the South Pacific; entering any elevator for a woman who was raped in an elevator).

Stimuli associated with the trauma are persistently avoided. The person commonly makes deliberate efforts to avoid thoughts, feelings, or conversations about the traumatic event (Criterion C1) and to avoid activities, situations, or people who arouse recollections of it (Criterion C2). This avoidance of reminders may include amnesia for an important aspect of the traumatic event (Criterion C3). Diminished responsiveness to the external world, referred to as "psychic numbing" or "emotional anesthesia", usually begins soon after the traumatic event. The individual may complain of having markedly diminished interest or participation in previously enjoyed activities (Criterion C4), of feeling detached or estranged from other people (Criterion C5), or having markedly reduced ability to feel emotions (especially those associated with intimacy, tenderness, and sexuality) (Criterion C6). The individual may have a sense of foreshortened future (e.g., not expecting to have a career, marriage, children, or a normal life span) (Criterion C7).

The individual has persistent symptoms of anxiety or increased arousal that were not present before the trauma. These symptoms may include falling or staying asleep that may be due to recurrent nightmares during which the traumatic event is relived (Criterion D1), hyper vigilance (Criterion D4), and exaggerated startle response (Criterion D5). Some individuals report irritability or outbursts of anger (Criterion D2) or difficulty concentrating or completing tasks (Criterion D3)."

Of notable interest in the DSM-IV diagnostic features of posttraumatic stress disorder is that they link the likelihood of posttraumatic stress disorders to the "intensity of and physical proximity to the stressor"; compare with PIE-model on

6

page 1 (American Psychiatric Association, 1994: p 424). No mention is made of the individual's pre-morbid functioning as being a probable contributor or predisposing factor in the onset of posttraumatic stress disorder.

Up till today no study has supplied data that demonstrated that a traumatic event has a greater formative effect than the predisposing pre-morbid factors (McFarlane, 1989).

A study of the literature indicates that the criteria of the DSM-IV do not explain the subjective predisposition to PTSD (Brewin, Andrews and Valentine, 2000; Yehuda and McFarlane, 1995). McFarlane (1989) reports that the incidence of PTSD at any given traumatic incident is rarely greater than 50%. This necessitates an explanation. Laposa and Alden (2001) states that PTSD is classified as an anxiety disorder, and typically with anxiety the person fears an impending threat, yet with PTSD, the event has already occurred, yet the patient behaves as though a past event is an impending event.

In a possible answer to this dilemma Ehlers and Clark (2000), proposed a cognitive model in which they assert that persistent PTSD occurs when people process the traumatic event in ways that lead to a sense of current, serious threat.

This sense of threat arises as result of:

1. inordinately negative appraisals of the trauma and its sequalae, and
2. disturbances in autobiographical memory

The latter points beg the question of personality traits. Clark, Watson and Mineka (1994) reviewed the literature on personality and stress disorders. They concluded that personality can affect PTSD in various ways and these may not be mutually exclusive:

- Personality can affect the individuals vulnerability to develop PTSD
- Personality characteristics can affect the course of expression of PTSD
- Personality can be affected by the experience of PTSD

It would rather seem that a complicated interaction of current stresses and pre-morbid factors in a person's subjective reality would create a unique probability of him/her experiencing such a condition.

1.4   Vicarious trauma: definition, etiology and description

Research studies by various authors indicate that emergency rescue workers, who are exposed to critical incidents on a cumulative basis, are at risk of incurring vicarious trauma. A critical incident can be defined as a traumatic event that occurs specifically in an occupational or occupational-related setting (Frolkey,1992).

Examples of Critical Incidents according to Mitchell (1988, p. 45) are:

1. The serious injury or death to children
2. Serious injury or death of a colleague
3. Serious injury or death to a female patient and/or death of a mother leaving small children behind
4. Suicide involving a fellow worker
5. Any disaster situation
6. Events where the victims are friends or family of the rescuer
7. Any event that seriously affects the lives of emergency personnel

8. Serious injury to an employee in the line of duty

McCann and Pearlman (1990) define vicarious trauma as the cumulative negative transformative effect on the helper of working with survivors of traumatic life events. This transformation involves gradual changes in the emergency rescue worker's view and experience of themselves, others and the world. This will be discussed later in more detail in terms of McCann & Pearlman's Constructivist Self-Developmental Theory.

According to McCammon, Durham, Jackson Alison and Williamson (1987) rescue workers may present with the following vicarious trauma symptoms:

- Repeated recollections of event
- Anhedonism
- Sadness
- Dreams of event
- Depression
- Being bothered by publicity
- Trying not to feel deeply
- Loss of enthusiasm
- Low morale
- Fatigue
- Guilt feelings
- Sense that event is recurring
- Frightening dreams of event
- General loss of interest
- Loss of appetite
- Startling easily
- Sleep disturbance
- Difficulty concentrating

- Detachment from people
- Avoiding activities that recall
- Trouble recalling things
- Loss of sexual desire

Of these, recollection and sadness seemed to be the most frequently endorsed symptoms.

1.4.1 Aetiology of vicarious trauma

In order to formulate a treatment plan for the sufferers of any form of pathology it is necessary to understand the dynamics and aetiology of that pathology. With regards to vicarious trauma, McFarlane refers to research by Clayton and Darvish (1979) citing former psychiatric illness as *"the only predictor of persistent depressive symptoms at 13 months"* (McFarlane, 1989, p.226). This finding was supported by Helzer, Robins and Wish (1979). In his own research McFarlane concluded that pre-morbid factors were more relevant to the condition of vicarious trauma than acute trauma.

Weiss, Marmar, Metzler and Ronfeldt (1995) and Marmar, Weiss, Metzler and Delucchi (1996) found that identifying individuals prone to peritraumatic dissociation during critical incident exposure was a strong predictor to vicarious trauma. Marmar et al (1996) concluded that rescue workers who are: shy, inhibited, insecure in their identity, portray poor leadership qualities, a tendency to irrational cognition's, belief fate is determined beyond their control and who cope with acute trauma through suppression, are at higher risk for acute disassociation responses to critical incidents. Immediate disassociation responses to trauma include feelings of detachment, derealisation, depersonalisation and out of body experiences.

In terms of a cognitive model Thompson and Suzuki (1991) reported that emergency rescue workers reported intrusive memories of work-related trauma. Clohessy and Ehlers (1999) indicated that negative interpretations of former recollections were predictive of vicarious trauma. Such negative interpretations correlate with Marmar's referral to irrational thought patterns.

Schnurr, Friedman and Rosenberg (1993) found in a study of men tested with the MMPI in college, reported that veterans who developed Posttraumatic Stress Disorder as a consequence of their Vietnam service had significantly high scores on the following scales:

- Hypochondriasis
- Psychopathic deviate
- Masculinity-femininity, and
- Paranoia scales than those who did not.

This group were generally less happy, more withdrawn and socially inhibited than their peers during college.

Based on these results, Marmar et al (1996) predict that emergency rescue workers with characteristics reflecting better adjustment, greater ambition, greater prudence, and stronger identity and sense of control could experience less dissociation at times of critical incident exposures.

High-risk candidates of vicarious trauma were identified by the following traits:

1. Overestimation of risk
2. Shyness
3. Inhibition
4. Uncertainty about their identity

5. Reluctance to take leadership roles
6. Global intuitive cognitive styles
7. Believe that fate and circumstances beyond their control determine their future
8. Cope with adversity by attempting to "sweep the problems under the rug" engaging in wishful thinking and suppress emotions rather than confront problems

They recommend that these individuals need to be screened out or be provided with additional training in recognising and coping with critical incident stress.

1.5 Secondary Traumatic Stress Disorder/ Compassion Fatigue

Secondary Traumatic Stress Disorder (STSD) can be described as the sudden adverse reactions emergency rescue staff can have to trauma survivors whom they assist or want to help (Jenkins and Baird, 2002).

Charles Figley (1983) first defined STSD as the emotional duress experienced by individuals having close contact with a trauma survivor, especially concerned family members, a natural response to a survivor's traumatic material with which emergency staff may identify or empathise (Figley and Kleber, 1995).

The symptoms of STSD are nearly identical to that of PTSD (see Table 1.1).

Table 1.1:   Traumatic Symptoms of Primary and Secondary Traumatic Stress
             Disorder

(PRIMARY) PTSD STRESSORS	(SECONDARY) COMPASSION FATIGUE STRESSORS
A. Experienced an event outside the range of usual human experiences that would be markedly distressing to almost anyone, an event such as rape, terrorism attacks, and other terrifying experiences.	Experienced indirectly the primary traumatic stressors through helping those who had experienced these traumas: helping in such roles as a nurse, social worker, fire fighter, paramedic, or other roles and activities.
B. Traumatic event is persistently re-experienced in one (or more) of the following ways:	Traumatic event is persistently re-experienced in one (or more) of the following ways:
1. Recurrent and intrusive distressing recollections of the event, including images, thoughts, or perceptions.	Recurrent and intrusive distressing recollections of the client/event, including images, thoughts, or perceptions.
2. Recurrent distressing dreams of the event.	Recurrent distressing dreams of the client/event
3. Acting or feeling as if the event were recurring (includes a sense of reliving the experience, illusions, hallucinations, and dissociative flashback episodes, including those that occur on awakening or when intoxicated.	Acting or feeling as if he traumatic event were recurring (includes a sense of reliving contact with the client and the client's story in order to solve the puzzle and help the client).
4. Intense psychological distress at exposure to internal or external cues that symbolize or resemble an aspect of the traumatic event.	Intense psychological distress at exposure to internal or external cues that symbolize or resemble the aspect of the work of helping others

5. Physiological reactivity on exposure to trauma cues	Physiological reactivity on exposure to trauma cues that are associated with the role of the helper
C. Persistent avoidance of stimuli associated with the trauma and numbing of general responsiveness (not present before the trauma), as indicated by three or more of the following:	Persistent avoidance of stimuli associated with the trauma and numbing of general responsiveness (not present before the trauma), as indicated by three or more of the following:
1. Efforts to avoid thoughts, feelings, or conversations associated with the trauma	Efforts to avoid thoughts, feelings, or conversations associated with the client's trauma
2. Efforts to avoid activities, places or people that arouse recollections of the trauma	Efforts to avoid activities, places, or people that arouse recollections of the client's trauma
3. Inability to recall an important aspect of the trauma	Errors in judgement about conceptualizing and treating the trauma case
4. Markedly diminished interest or participation in significant activities	Markedly diminished interest or participation in significant activities
5. Feeling of detachment or estrangement from others	Feeling of detachment or estrangement from others
6. Restricted range of affect (e.g. unable to have loving feelings)	Restricted range of affect (e.g. unable to know the client personally or saviour orientated)
7. Sense of foreshortened future (e.g. does not expect to have a career, marriage, children, or normal lifespan)	Sense of foreshortened future (e.g. does not expect or want long career)
D. Persistent symptoms of increased arousal (not present before the trauma), as indicated by two or more of the following:	Persistent symptoms of increased arousal (not present before the trauma), as indicated by two or more of the following:

1. Difficulty falling or staying asleep	Difficulty falling or staying asleep
2. Irritability or outbursts of anger	Irritability or outbursts of anger
3. Difficulty concentrating	Difficulty concentrating
4. Hypervigilance	Hypervigilance
5. Exaggerated startle response	Exaggerated startle response
E. 30 days duration	30 days duration
F. Disturbance causes significant distress or impairment in social, occupational, or other important areas of functioning: Evidenced by increased family conflict, sexual dysfunction, poor interpersonal communication, less loving, more dependant, reduced social support, poor stress-coping methods	Disturbance causes clinically significant distress or impairment in social, occupational, or other important areas of functioning: Evidenced by increased work conflict, missed work, insensitivity to clients, lingering distress caused by trauma material, reduced social support, poor stress-coping methods

(Figley, 2003: p4-5)

The core difference is that the traumatised survivor may develop PTSD, whereas the person/ helper hearing about the trauma or assisting the survivor of the trauma may develop STSD. The onset of STSD can be sudden and without warning, and is related more to the traumas experienced by clients and or significant others rather than occupational stress itself (Saben-Farrell and Turnip, 2003).

Figley has now renamed the condition Compassion Fatigue, viewing it as a normative occupational hazard for trauma workers and explaining that the term is more preferable to STSD for being less stigmatising (Figley, 1995). More recently a burn-out component were incorporated to explain the energy draining characteristic of secondary trauma that represents the exhaustion of providing ongoing support to the chronically affected primary victim (Figley and Kleber, 1995).

There are three content domains of symptoms:

1. the re-experiencing of the primary survivor's traumatic event
2. avoidance of reminders and /or numbing in response to reminders
3. persistent arousal both emotionally and somatically

Sabin-Farrell and Turpin (2003) suggest that additional important elements associated with this construct are:

-   cognitive changes in beliefs and attitudes; and
-   additional effects on interpersonal and occupational functioning.

1.6 Burnout

The construct of burnout is far better developed in theory than the former two trauma constructs. It was first used by psychologists in occupational stress literature to describe and explain emotional consequences which are specific human service workers and mental health professionals who work with other people's problems (Maslach, 1987).

Burnout is conceptualised as a defensive response to prolonged occupational exposure to demanding interpersonal situations that produce psychological strain and provide inadequate support. Maslach (1982) defines burnout as containing three content domains:

"A syndrome of emotional exhaustion, depersonalization, and reduced personal accomplishment that can occur among individuals who do people- work of some kind… response to the chronic emotional strain of dealing extensively with other human beings, particularly when they are troubled or having problems… a pattern of emotional overload and subsequent emotional exhaustion is at the heart of the burnout syndrome. A person gets overly involved emotionally, overextends him-/herself, and feels overwhelmed by the emotional demands imposed by other people"(p.3).

Although the three components are conceptually distinct, they are not assumed to be empirically uncorrelated since they share the same causes (Jackson, Schwab and Schuler, 1986).

1.7 Comparing Secondary Trauma, Vicarious Trauma, and Burnout

Secondary Trauma, Vicarious Trauma and Burnout are similar in resulting from exposure to emotionally charged and engaging clients. They represent debilitation that can impair the providers' services (Jenkins and Baird, 2002).

Burnout occurs as a result of any kind of prolonged tedious work, and focuses on symptoms of emotional exhaustion resulting from job strain, erosion of idealism, and a reduced sense of accomplishment and achievement (Figley, 1995; Maslach, 1982).

Vicarious Trauma and Secondary Trauma occurs, not as result of workplace conditions (as burnout) but as result of specific exposure to traumatised clients.

Vicarious Trauma and Secondary Trauma also differ in four ways (Jenkins & Baird, 2002):

1) Focus on symptomatology vs. theory
   Figley (1995) focuses on observed PTSD symptomatology vs. McCann &Pearlman (1990) and Pearlman and Saakvitne (1995) emphasising the theoretical foundation of VT as a process of self-perceived change.

2) Nature of symptoms (observable reactions vs. covert cognitive changes)
   Figley (1995) focuses on PTSD symptoms with rapid onset as central, yet acknowledges trauma-related cognitive shifts. McCann and Pearlman (1990) recognise PTSD symptoms, but emphasise their content rather than intensity in the context of profound belief system changes.

3) <u>Relevant populations</u>

Figley (1995) expanded his concept to apply to professionals who provide services to all trauma survivors. McCann and Pearlman (1990) and Pearlman and Saakvitne (1995) have focused on mental health professionals who primarily work with survivors of incest and childhood sexual abuse.

4) <u>Amount of exposure to trauma survivors</u>

Figley (1995) concluded that only one severe exposure to one particular person's trauma can result in secondary traumatic symptoms. McCann and Pearlman (1990) argue that VT results from cumulative exposure to traumatised clients over time.

CHAPTER TWO

THEORETICAL MODELS

2.1   Introduction

A cognitive-behavioural theory of PTSD which focuses on factors that maintain the latter, were developed by Williams (1999). Drawing on Beck's concept of dysfunctional assumptions, it is suggested that negative attitudes to emotional states and their expression could lead to avoidant tendencies that block the processing of traumatic information. This is an elaboration of Horowitz's model.

Horowitz (1986) proposed that, subsequent to a traumatic episode, there is an initial outcry or stunned reaction followed by a period of information overload, in which thoughts, memories and images of the trauma cannot be reconciled with current schemata. Accordingly various psychological defense mechanisms come into operation to keep traumatic information unconscious and the individual experiences a period of denial. Completion tendencies, however, help to keep the trauma information in active memory, causing it to break trough these defenses and intrude into consciousness in the form of flashbacks, nightmares, and unwanted thoughts as the person attempts to merge the trauma information with existing models.

This tension between completion tendency and the psychological defense mechanisms causes survivors to oscillate between phases of intrusion and denial-numbing as they integrate the traumatic material with their long-term schematic representations (Horowitz, 1986).

Laposa and Alden's (2001) research results supported the importance of cognitive processes in PTSD. Negative appraisals of the event were predictive of more intense PTSD symptoms, i.e. the way in which the persons interpreted these recollections had implications for the severity of PTSD symptoms. Ehlers and Steil (1995) observed that people differ in the meaning that they assign to the occurrence and content of intrusive recollections of traumatic events. Some may interpret them as a normal part of recovery from a traumatic event. Others interpret them in a more negative way, for example as an indication of weakness or an indication that they are going mad.

Such negative interpretations are important in explaining the maintenance of intrusive recollections and PTSD in general because they determine:

- How distressing the intrusions are
- The extent to which the person engages in strategies to control the intrusions and then prevent change in meaning of the trauma and posttraumatic intrusions.

Williams, Hodgkinson, Joseph and Yule (1995) found that a higher endorsement of dysfunctional attitudes as assessed were associated with higher scores on some symptoms. It was argued that the subjects' attitude to emotion reflects a maintenance factor rather than an onset mechanism. Survivors with more negative attitudes also received less social support which would correlate with a poorer recovery rate.

The latter forms part of Janoff-Bulman's (1985) cognitive appraisal theory that states: PTSD is the result of the destruction of certain basic assumptions about the world, namely:
- The assumption of personal invulnerability
- The perception of the world as being meaningful and comprehensible
- View one-self in a positive light

Although numerous theories exist on PTSD (see discussion in 1.3) only two theoretical models will be discussed in this paper. The reason for this is that for the purpose of this research the two models discussed are the only two found, in an extensive research of the literature, that specifically attempt to explain the phenomena of Secondary traumatic stress/compassion fatigue and/or vicarious trauma.

The first model called the: **Constructivist Self Developmental Theory** was co-authored by Laurie Pearlman and Lisa McCann in 1990. The model blends contemporary psychoanalytic theory (self-psychology and object relations theory) with social cognition theories to provide a developmental framework for understanding the experiences of survivors of traumatic events, specifically vicarious trauma (Pearlman and Mac Ian, 1995).

Constructivist Self Developmental Theory (CSDT) observes individuals' adjustments to trauma as interactions between their own personalities (defensive styles, psychological needs and coping styles) and prominent aspects of the traumatic events, all in the framework of social and cultural variables that shape psychological reactions (Pearlman and Mac Ian, 1995).

The second theoretical model that will be discussed is the: **Theory of Survival Strategies** developed by Paul Valent in 1995. The theory attempts to heuristically explain the wide variety of symptoms of secondary trauma/compassion fatigue, that are relived or avoided after trauma, and why they should be experienced.

Figley (1995) suggested that PTSD should be called primary posttraumatic stress disorder and that similar symptoms experienced by helpers of trauma victims be called secondary traumatic stress disorder (STSD). The only differences between PTSD and STSD being (according to Figley) that: the latter resulted out of exposure to the trauma victims or their ordeal, and not the traumatic event itself.

Secondly that the intrusion and avoidance symptoms concerned the primary victims experience and not the helpers' own.

As PTSD as a diagnostic category is inadequate in explaining the wide variety of symptoms, STSD does not heuristically define and unite the wide variety of symptoms as mentioned before (Table I.1).

Counter transference may explain the means of transmission of symptoms and reason for suffering. It is described as the unconscious awareness to and absorption of survivors' symptoms of trauma. Yet, transference responses do not explain why particular symptoms should be transmitted at any particular time (Valent, 2003).

Burnout may be one reason for a particular cluster of symptoms. The phenomena is characterised by certain psychological arousal symptoms, such as headaches, pessimism, and cynicism, problems in work relations, poor work performance, interpersonal conflict, irritability, aggression, as well as mental and physical exhaustion.

The former condition can occur as result of the potential harmful nature of work stresses or managerial pressures, constraints, or lack of empathy. Yet it does not explain why they should occur during secondary traumatic stress and others not, nor does it explain the prevalence of symptoms outside this particular cluster.

Other explanations for the character of symptoms reside in survival strategies such as fight or flight. These are however equally inadequate to give sufficient reasons the diversity of symptoms.

2.2 Constructivist Self Developmental Theory (CSDT)

There seems to be a significant relationship between 1) traumatic life events, 2) cognitive schemas about self and the world, and 3) psychological adaptation. This model has been elaborated into a theory of personality called the constructivist self-development theory (CSDT) by McCann and Pearlman (1990). The theory emphasises adaptation and the active construction to meaning.

Symptoms of trauma are viewed as adaptations to events. Adaptations are based on the context in which an event occurs and it's meaning to the individual. CSDT assumes that "irrational" or distorted beliefs reflect an attempt to protect one-self and one's meaning system from the harm that trauma threatens.

CSDT aspects of the self impacted by psychological trauma are:

1. Frame of reference
2. Self capacities
3. Ego resources
4. Psychological needs and cognitive resources
5. Memory and perception

2.2.1. Frame of reference

The self includes frame of reference: the underlying sense of identity, worldview, and spirituality that informs the individual's perception of himself, his world, his relationships, and his experiences. Combined, these beliefs create the lens through which a person subjectively views the world and interprets their experiences (Saakvitne and Pearlman, 1992).

It also involves cognitive processes of causality and attribution. Any disruptions in an established frame of reference, e.g. the belief that the world is generally a safe place, can cause disorientation for the rescue worker and adversely affect their empathy for trauma survivors (Trippany, White Kress and Allan Wilcoxon, 2004).

2.2.2. Self capacities

An individual's experience of self is strongly shaped by their capacities for inner balance, specifically capacities to:

- Manage strong feelings
- To feel entitled to be alive and deserving of love
- To hold on to an inner awareness of caring for others.

These self-capacities influence how someone understands and integrates significant events in their lives and their value perceptions on them. An example would be a person's ability to self-soothe and maintain a sense of inner equilibrium.

Vicarious trauma may result in rescue workers experiencing a loss of identity, interpersonal difficulties, and difficulty controlling negative emotions or avoiding exposure to media that conveys the suffering of others, or feeling unable to meet the needs of loved one's in their lives (Trippany et al, 2004).

2.2.3. Ego resources

An important part of the self is the individual's abilities to negotiate interpersonal situations and to make appropriate decisions. These are referred to as ego resources. They include skills in self-awareness, willpower, initiative and striving for personal growth. Ego resources also include skills in interpersonal relationships, including foresight, self-protective judgements and the establishment of self-protective boundaries.

Disruption of these ego resources may lead to symptoms of perfectionism, and overextension at work. Rescue workers may also experience an inability to empathise with trauma survivors (Trippany et al, 2004).

2.2.4. Cognitive schemas and psychological needs

The cognitive portion of the theory is built upon a constructivist foundation; namely that human beings construct their own personal realities through the development of complex cognitive structures which are used to interpret events. These cognitive structures become increasingly more complex over the life span as individuals interact with their meaningful environment.

According to Piaget (1971) these cognitive structures (referred to as schemas) include beliefs, assumptions, and expectations about self and the world that enable individuals to make sense of their experience. Examples of such schemas are beliefs and assumptions about causality, the trustworthiness of sensory data, identity, and the self-world relations (Mahoney, 1981).

McCann and Pearlman (1990) reveal five fundamental psychological needs:

(i) Safety

A sense of security is basic to safety needs. Rescue workers experiencing vicarious trauma may feel that there is no safe haven to protect them from real or imagined threats to personal safety. Pearlman and Saakvitne (1995) suggests that higher levels of fearfulness, vulnerability, and concern may be ways in which this disruption in needs of safety is displayed.

(ii) Esteem

Esteem here refers to the need to view other people as kind, caring and therefore worthy of respect. People who are victims of trauma through the malevolent acts of other people (either single or multiple) may experience reduced esteem for other human beings. Rescue workers who experience vicarious trauma may be struggling with the discrepancy between their own positive schemas about human beings and the reality of the terrible abuses that people commit. They may experience a sense of anger at other people and the world in general as they contemplate on the potential evilness of others (McCann and Pearlman, 1990).

(iii) Trust/dependency

Through working with the victims of violence, emergency rescue workers may find that their schemas regarding trust are disrupted. During a phase of vicarious trauma they may become suspicious of other people's motives, more cynical, or distrustful (McCann and Pearlman, 1990).

(iv) Control

Persons, who are victims of trauma, often present with symptoms of helplessness and defencelessness. Rescue workers who are confronted with these situations may become concerned about their own sense of control and efficiency in the world. Rescue workers who are keen on being in control, may start fantasising about how they would protect their own family in such a situation. These fantasies may at times be violent or castigatory, articulating their need to reiterate their belief in their own power (McCann and Pearlman, 1990).

Rescue workers may experience a diminished sense of liberty in terms of movement and self-governance. Over identification with their clients may lead to nightmares in which they are trapped or confined. This may become dysfunctional if it were to lead to inappropriate attempts to control others or excessive anger about one's in ability to do so (McCann and Pearlman, 1990).

(v) Intimacy

Survivors of trauma often experience a sense of alienation from the world and others. Rescue workers who are exposed to such individuals' horrific experiences may, themselves, experience a sense of estrangement. The latter condition may be aggravated by other professionals who regard the work that they do with repugnance.

As victims of trauma may feel ashamed by their experience (survivor guilt or a suppressed sense of sorrow for not having done enough to prevent the event occurring), rescue workers may equally experience a sense of detachment from their colleagues, family, friends and partners/spouses, believing that they would not be able to empathise and understand what they are experiencing. Ethical issues of client confidentiality may further deepen the sense of alienation for the rescue workers (McCann and Pearlman, 1990).

The cognitive manifestations of psychological needs are schemas. McCann and Pearlman's (1990) major hypothesis is that **trauma can disrupt these schemas**. The unique way in which the trauma is experienced depends in part upon which schemas are central for the individual. At the time of a traumatic experience each person will adapt and cope given their current context(s) and early experiences: interpersonal, intra-psychic, familial, cultural, and social.

A second hypothesis is that **individuals who work with trauma survivors, i.e. emergency rescue workers, can also find that their schemas are adversely affected** in these areas. Their unique reactions will be determined by the centrality of these schemas to themselves.

2.2.5. Memory and perception

Memory and perception are complex and multimodal. Any experience is processed and recalled through several modalities including (Trippany et al, 2004):

- Verbal memory (cognitive narrative)
- Visual (pictures stored in the mind)
- Affective (emotions experienced)
- Somatic /sensory (physical sensations)
- Interpersonal (resulting dynamics in current interpersonal relationships)

A non-fragmented memory is encoded along all these dimensions, which are integrated and interconnected, i.e. a memory (schemata) of a particular event will include many of these modalities of memory.

Traumatic memories often involve the dissociation or disconnection of different aspects of the experience, resulting in fragmentation e.g., the narrative may be recalled without feelings or images (Saakvitne and Pearlman, 1992). This will happen in an effort of the fight-or-flight mechanism (situated in the hypothalamus-pituitary-adrenal axis) to protect the individual from the full horror of the traumatic event.

Like the trauma victim, rescue workers may experience their clients' traumatic imagery recurring as fragments without content or connotation. They may occur as flashbacks, dreams, or intrusive thoughts and could be seen as the hallmark of PTSD (McCann & Pearlman, 1990).

It is suggested that the most excruciating imagery centers around the schemas related to the rescue worker's most important need areas. Therefore, what is remembered in the imagery system of memory is tinted by schemas, which is encoded in verbal representation system of memory (Paivio, 1986).

Disruption in the imagery system of memory is often associated with potent emotional states (Bower, 1981; Paivio,1986). Rescue workers may experience feelings of anger, sadness and anger due to their work with victims of trauma. These feeling states may be activated within conscious awareness or be repressed out of conscious awareness. The latter may occur with rescue workers who are exposed to traumatic imagery that is too overwhelming, emotionally or cognitively to integrate.

The former theory can be summarized as follow:

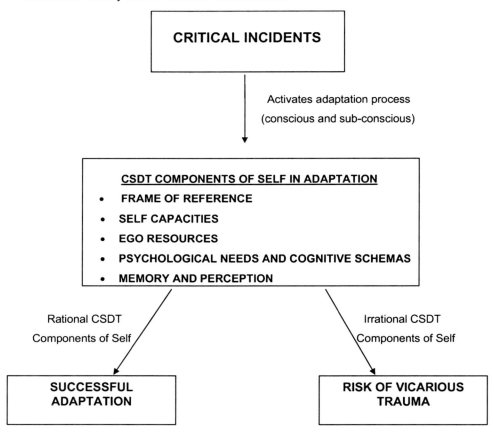

Figure 2.1 Constructivist Self Developmental Theory Diagram

2.3 Theory of Survival Strategies

The biological theories of traumatic stress disorder have evolved from both animal models of stress and from measures of biological variables in clinical populations with this disorder. From both sets of data many neurotransmitter systems have been concerned. Preclinical models of learned helplessness, provocation, and sensitization in animals have led to theories about nor epinephrine, dopamine, endogenous opioids, and benzodiazepine receptors and the hypothalamic-pituitary-adrenal axis (Kaplan and Sadock, 1998).

In clinical populations data have supported hypotheses that the noradrenergic and endogenous opiate systems, as well as the hypothalamus-pituitary-adrenal axis are hyperactive in at least some patients with PTSD. Other biological findings of significance are increased activity and responsiveness of the autonomic nervous system, as substantiated by elevated heart rates and blood pressure readings as well as by abnormal sleep patterns (Kaplan and Sadock, 1998).

Hagh-Shenas, Goldstein, and Yule (1999) suggest specific hemispheric involvement in the processing of trauma associated information as opposed to mere unpleasant information. This may partially be linked to the bias of the right hemisphere in processing emotionally laden material, suggesting that in times of trauma occurring, without the opportunity for any processing of it, the right hemisphere preferentially mediates the information, consequently storing it in a predominantly non-verbal form. Therapy would then attempt to convert these schemas into verbal structures that are then open to treatment.

Valent (2003) describes survival strategies as being "bio-psychosocial templates" that have developed to promote greatest possible continued existence within evolutionary social units. They function in the "old mammalian" (hypothalamus-pituitary-adrenal axis) brain between instincts and abstract functioning. During traumatic situations, they correspond to acute stress responses.

31

PTSD arousal symptoms suggest that only fight and flight acute stress symptoms are relived and avoided. Valent (2003) proposes that six other such survival strategies are part to reliving and avoidance responses.

The eight survival strategies proposed by Valent (2003) are:

1. Rescuing (Caretaking)
2. Attaching
3. Asserting (Goal achieving)
4. Adapting (Goal surrender)
5. Fighting
6. Fleeing
7. Competing
8. Cooperating

Valent states that it is their adaptive, maladaptive, biological, psychological and social components that contribute to the extensive myriad of symptoms in STSD (see Table 2.1). Survival strategies and their mechanisms are elements of a dynamic process. They are activated by personal judgments of stressors with which they are supposed to cope. When they are unsuccessful, it may result in trauma and illness. This effect may be alleviated by defense mechanisms and retrograde amnesia of the trauma.

SUCCESSFUL / ADAPTIVE RESPONSES					UNSUCCESSFUL / MALADAPTIVE RESPONSES			
APPRAISAL OF MEANS OF SURVIVAL	SURVIVAL STRATEGIES	BIOLOGICAL	PSYCHOLOGICAL	SOCIAL	BIOLOGICAL	PSYCHOLOGICAL	SOCIAL	TRAUMA RESPONSES
Must save others	Rescuing Protect Provide	↑ Estrogen ↑ Oxytocin ↑ Opioids	Care Empathy **Devotion**	Responsibility Nurture **Preservation**	Sympathetic & Parasymp. Arousal	Burden Depletion **Self-concern**	Resentment Neglect **Rejection**	Anguish Compass Fatigue Caused death
Must be saved by others	Attaching Protected Provided	? ↑Opioids	Held, cared for Nurtured **Looked after**	Close, secure Content **Union**	↑ Opioids	Yearning Need crave **Abandonment**	Cry insecure Deprived **Separation**	Helplessness Cast out Left to die
Must achieve goal	Asserting Combat Work	↑ E, NE ↓ Cortisol ↑ Immunocomp	Strength Control **Potency**	Will High morale **Success**	↑↑ E, NE Depletion E, NE ↑ BP, ? CHD	Frustration Loss of control **Impotence**	Willfulness Low morale **Failure**	Exhaustion "Burn-out" Powerlessness
Must surrender goal	Adapting Accept Grieve	Parasymp Arousal ↑ Cortisol	Acceptance Sadness, grief **Hope**	Yielding Mourning **Turn to new**	↑ Cortisol ↓ Immunocomp ↑ Infection, ? ↑ CA	Overwhelmed Depression **Despair**	Collapsed Withdrawal **Giving up**	Damaged Given in Succumbing
Must remove danger	Fighting Defend Rid	Symp. Arousal ↑N, NE ↑ BP	Threat Revenge **Frighten**	Deterrence Wounding **Riddance**	↑↑ Symp Arousal ↓ Cortisol	Hatred Persecution **Killing**	Attack Eradication **Destruction**	Horror Evil Murder
Must remove oneself from danger	Fleeing Run, hide, save oneself	Sympathetic & Parasymp Arousal	Fear Terror **Deliverance**	Retreat Flight **Escape**	NE depletion ↑ E & Cortisol	Phobia Paranoia **Engulfment**	Avoidance Panic **Annihilation**	"Inescapable shock" Being hunted Killed
Must obtain scarce essentials	Competing Power Acquisition	↑Testosterone Symp. Arousal	Winning Status **Dominance**	Contest Hierarchy **Possession**	↓ Testosterone ↓ Female Horms ↑ Cortisol	Defeat Greed, Envy **Exploitation**	Oppression Struggle **Plunder**	Terrorization Marginalization Elimination
Must create more essentials	Cooperating Trust Mutual gain	↑ Opiates ↓BP, E, NE	Mutuality Generosity Love	Integration Reciprocity Creativity	↓ Opiates ? ↑ Parasymp Arousal	Betrayal Selfishness **Abuse**	Disconnection Cheating **Disintegration**	Fragmentation Alienation Decay

Notes for Table 2: E = epinephrine. NE = norepinephrine. Immunocomp = immunocompetence. Parasymp. = parasympathetic (nervous system). Symp = sympathetic (nervous system). BP = blood pressure. CHD = coronary heart disease. CA = cancer. Compass = compassion (Valent, 2003 pp.22-23).

Table 2.1   Valent's

Survival Strategies

Valent argues that secondary traumatic stress (a less serious, more acute form of STSD) and secondary traumatic stress disorder are the result of counter transference identification with victims' maladaptive and traumatic aspects of helpers' survival strategies respectively, and/or one's own complimentary survival strategies being insufficient to various degrees (p.25, 2003).

He reasons that compassion fatigue and burnout are specific failed Rescue-Caretaking and Assertiveness-Goal Achievement survival strategy responses. They are prominent in rescue workers because they are usually corresponding to victim needs.

2.3.1 Secondary Traumatic Stress and Counter Transference Responses

Maladaptive (stress) responses in Table 2.1 are referred to as secondary traumatic stress responses and are induced in rescue workers by means of a combined association with victim survival strategies with that of their own. Through association, the rescue worker empathizes with the victim and is more vigilant to warning signs and the individual's requirements. Counter transference occurs between the rescue worker and the victim, as the rescue worker re-experience the event within themselves thus enhancing comprehension for the victim's distress.

The significance of counter transference is to instigate adaptive survival strategies within the rescue worker that would compensate for and strengthen incapable victims. For example, an individual in panic (maladaptive Flight) may be offered a getaway and freedom (adaptive Flight); overwhelmed people (maladaptive Competition) may be empowered and offered rank (adaptive Competition); neglected, deprived people (maladaptive Attachment) may be offered care and support (adaptive Rescue-Caretaking); lack of ability to grieve (Adaptation-Goal Surrender) may be aided empathy and optimism.

Rescue workers' survival strategies are often the adaptive equal of the victims' maladaptive strategies, or the adaptive equivalents of the adjoining reciprocal survival strategies (see Table 2.1), or modified aspects of broad ranging survival strategies.

Valent (2003) accordingly makes states the following conclusions:

- Counter transference, although widely accepted in long-term psychotherapy, has the ability to cause significant impact in acute situations.
- When rescue workers' survival strategies are inadequate to cope with victim stresses, they become secondarily stressed by the burden of both the transference of the victims' maladaptive survival strategies as well as their own maladaptive balancing survival strategies.
- During critical incidents all survival strategies may be activated, therefore rescue workers may experience all survival strategies to some degree.
- Both rescue workers as well as victims of trauma experience adaptive and maladaptive survival strategies. Helpers may therefore not only be stressed by critical incidents, but also fulfilled (compare Frankl's logo therapy for victims of the Holocaust).

2.3.2 Secondary Traumatic Stress Disorder

Secondary traumatic stress disorder (STSD) occurs in correspondence to secondary traumatic stress. Therefore rescue workers may experience STSD through over-identifying with the trauma victims' reactions (see Table 2.1) or their own dysfunctional matching efforts may reach critical proportions.

For example, a rescue worker may respond to a victim's cries of help but not be able to save the person. Accordingly the helper's STSD may include both identification with unavoidable distress and horror of imminent destruction (trauma of Flight) of the victim, and his own compassion fatigue (trauma of Rescue).

2.3.3 Compassion Strain and Fatigue

By understanding of the survival strategy Rescue-Caretaking allows, according to Valent (2003) for an exploratory distinction of compassion stress and compassion fatigue from the more general secondary traumatic stress and STSD.

Table 2.1 demonstrates that the judgment of rescue workers that they need to rescue or assist others ignites Rescue-Caretaking responses. The psychological and social components of these responses are:

- Care
- Empathy
- Devotion
- Responsibility
- Nurture
- Perseveration

Combined these responses act as the mechanism of compassion stress can be viewed in the unsuccessful, maladaptive psychological and social responses of Rescue-Caretaking. They are:

- A sense of burden
- Depletion and self concern
- Resentment
- Neglect
- Rejection

In rescue workers these feelings culminate into strain, stress and distress. Compassion stress can be aggravated by explicit negative psychosocial feedback judgments (for example being irresponsible in the Judgments column in Table 2.1) and by emerging meanings bout one's poor role, failed expectations and human limitations.

When victims of trauma could not be successfully rescued or treated, compassion strain may reach traumatic proportions and may be called compassion fatigue. It would include maladaptive compassion strain, but in addition includes severe distress and intense guilt regarding not having been able to prevent or perhaps even causing harm or death.

The term compassion can also be applied to a profound sympathy and sorrow for those affected by suffering and sorrow, specifically as responses for those in grief (Adaptation-Goal Surrender). Other specific words mentioned by Valent are:

- Pity for refugees (Flight)
- Support for the helpless (Attachment)
- Tenderness for the abused (Cooperation).

2.3.4 Burnout

Burnout according to Valent (2003) can be related to the survival strategy Assertiveness-Goal Achievement. As goals are being achieved rescue workers may believe that they are enforcing their will and accordingly feel:

- Strong
- In control
- Powerful
- High morale
- Successful

Failure to accomplish goals may be accompanied by:

- Frustration
- A sense of loss of control
- Powerlessness
- Increased unyielding efforts
- Diminished morale

Numerous burnout symptoms such as: poor work performance, irritability, poor concentration are resulting from the symptoms mentioned above. Work stress increase sympathetic nervous symptoms listed in Table 2.1, which then produces general burnout symptoms such as sleep difficulties, muscle tension, hypertension, coronary disease and stroke.

Traumatic intensities of Assertiveness contain earlier burnout symptoms as well as intense exhaustion and helplessness.

2.3.5 Diagnosis of helper stress

In summery compassion stress and fatigue, as well as burnout stress and fatigue are stress and trauma responses in two specific survival strategies:

- Rescue-Caretaking and,
- Assertiveness-Goal Achievement.

Trauma symptoms in emergency rescue workers appear in different forms at different times in the secondary traumatic process (see Table 2.1). Symptoms of trauma occur due to the failure of survival strategies, whereas symptoms of stress occur due to ineffective or maladaptive survival strategies (Valent, 2003).

Every time stress, trauma symptoms may be classified as biological, psychological and social aspects of specific survival strategies. They can be drawn back to indemnificatory or supplementary survival strategies in particular victim-helper interactions (Valent, 2003).

Similar to the reliving and avoidance symptoms of PTSD, rescue workers may experience intrusive secondary symptoms of stress or STSD. They may also present with defenses to avoid and diminish traumatic states, thoughts of guilt, shame, and shattered meanings. In these cases their recollections of the primary critical incident may be deficient or nor present at all.

Symptoms and illnesses are a consequence of relived or avoided biological, psychological, and social secondary stress and trauma symptoms. Survival strategies affix the core substance of what is re-experienced or avoided as well as its meaning.

2.4   Approach for treating Secondary Traumatic Stress Symptoms

2.4.1   Introduction

From the former two theoretical models it seems evident that critical incidents, alone, do not explain the origin of secondary traumatic stress symptoms, secondary traumatic stress disorder, compassion fatigue or vicarious trauma. Not all emergency rescue workers exposed to trauma will experience the same condition or symptoms at the same time. All depends on subjective differences in the processing and adjustment as previously discussed.

Subjective experiences/perceptions, both past and present, seem to be the hallmark of predicting possible secondary trauma symptoms in any situation in any person at any moment. From the literature it would seem sensible to emphasis subjective differences in the individual. This would accordingly make cultural and other macro differences predominately redundant in the explanation of etiology or treatment of secondary trauma symptoms/ conditions.

This begs the question what cluster of elements would add value to predicting the possibility and prognosis of secondary trauma symptoms/ diagnosis? It is proposed that, as in the case of PTSD, personality traits, and psycho-social history may contribute to etiology and or maintenance of secondary traumatic symptoms. It therefore seems appropriate that a personality (personalogical) based treatment approach would be most efficacious in the treatment of secondary stress symptoms with the emphasis on individual needs and individual capabilities.

Ever since the 1970's academic publications in the field of mental health, emergency services, and disaster management have contained reports and studies on the effects of trauma response work on the emergency rescue staff. During the eighties and nineties the focus in the literature was on the effects of trauma on firefighters, police officers, and emergency medical staff (Myers and Wee, 2003).

This period saw the emergence of professional publications on the management of secondary trauma stress symptoms as well as vicarious trauma symptoms. McCammon, Durham, Jackson-Alison and Williamson (1987) described the condition as a "disease of adaptation". They viewed the impact of disaster work to beat least temporarily stressful with the potential to lead to long-term psychological difficulties.

Since the 1960's consensus had been reached in the majority of publications that stress and therefore all critical incidents are in evitable aspects of life. It is the way one chooses to cope that largely defines the degree of successful adaptation. This can be based on the relationship between experiencing a difficult event and positive adjustment (McCammon et al, 1987).

2.4.2 Coping Strategies

The two critical processes which arbitrate this person-environment relationship, according to McCammon et al (1987), are:

- Cognitive appraisals, and
- Ways of coping.

It is therefore not the incident itself that determines people's response to it, but how one chooses to evaluate the stimulus and the consequential emotions it evokes. Lazarus and Folkman (1984) define the construct coping as the process with which people positively adapt to the demands and emotions generated by that which is appraised as stressful/traumatic. These processes of assessment and coping are not necessarily separate.

Moos and Schaeffer (1986) identified three areas of coping skills that influence trauma recovery:

1. **Appraisal-focused coping** entails interpreting the meaning in an incident through logical analysis, mental preparation, cognitive redefinition, and cognitive avoidance or denial.
2. **Problem-focused coping** involves the practical aspects of seeking information and support, taking action in terms of problem-solving and recognizing alternative rewards.
3. **Emotion-focused coping** deals with affective management, emotional discharge and reconciled acceptance.

Taylor (1983) identified three themes/goals in the adjustment process to traumatic events. They are:

1. **A search for meaning** in the experience, involving attempts to understand the incident, its cause and significance.
2. **An effort to gain mastery** over the incident, involving gaining control over the event and one's life, preventing similar events from re-occurring as well as strategies for controlling the current incident.
3. **Restoring self-esteem** through self-enhancing evaluations to find ways of feeling good about one-self, in spite of the oppressive event, which potentially can reduce self-esteem.

The shared quality of Taylor's themes is that they propose a phenomenological (subjective) approach in appraising the events/facts in such a way as to minimize negativity and accordingly potential risk of emotional contamination. A popular view in the literature is that people who view an incident as a challenge cope better than those who view it as a threat.

This raises the issue of active cognitive coping. Accordingly it was found by Moos and Billings (1982) that active cognitive coping, involving logical analysis and cognitive redefinition, correlates better with successful adaptation than avoidance strategies. Furthermore it was found that a diverse range of coping skills are more effective than single strategies.

2.4.3 Cognitions and Behaviors

In studies conducted by Durham, McCammon and Jackson Alison (1985) and McCammon et al (1987) the following cognitive approaches were identified among emergency rescue staff in two separate rescue projects, the one involving an explosion in an apartment building and secondly a tornado (see Table 2.2).

Some of the most frequently endorsed strategies were: compassion satisfaction, feeling satisfied in being able to help. The next most frequently endorsed strategy was to reframe the situation. Other cognitive coping strategies that were endorsed included using humor, realistically examining their fears, being thoughtful towards others. Due to the grand scale of the tornado rescue workers were inclined to look towards finding meaning and philosophical contemplation.

Although the frequently used traits point to cognitive strategies, tornado rescue staff were more inclined to make use of social support. The magnitude of an incident may therefore impact on the coping strategies utilized (McCammon et al, 1987).

Table 2.2. Frequency of Coping Behaviors used in Emergency Personnel

Coping Behavior	Frequency of use (%)		Behavior Helpful (%)	
	Explosion	*Tornado*	*Explosion*	*Tornado*
Remind self providing help		78		97
Remind self things could be worse	57	68	90	93
Look at situation realistically	53	68	92	89
Figure out things you feared really could have happened	48	30	70	89
Concentrate on other things	44	52	84	86
Think about humorous parts of event	42	56	85	79
Be more helpful to others	41	60	95	92
Think of meaning of life following event	38	54	94	93
Work on expectations for future	38	39	86	96
Let self experience all feelings about event	38	58	90	89
Talk to others about incident	38	64	96	86
Put feelings out of mind	32	45	72	91
Think about good things in life	32	45	87	78
Figure out when responses were irrational	30	42	78	91
Devote self to work	29	28	70	95
Figure out how things would be different if you acted on a different way	29	32	78	74
Seek out other workers dealing with same thing	25	42	84	86
Figure out meaning of being in rescue work	24	23	74	82
Put whole thing out of mind	23	32	66	86
Withdraw from people	20	37	82	88
Develop positive attitude about incident	19	33	82	93
Think about what happened alone	19	34	85	85
Figure out why disaster made you feel as it did	18	28	74	75
Not be bothered by conflicting feelings	17	19	65	92
Involve self in other activities	17	20	71	92
Seek increased emotional support from others	11	33	77	64
Look for someone to provide direction	11	17	76	58
Turn to religion or philosophy for help	10	26	78	46
Find new interests	6	11	48	57
Spend more time listening to music, writing or getting in touch with nature	6	14	68	43
Do things impulsively to see if such activities would help	5	10	55	38
Figure out choices in life and how they are related to the event	4	15	69	40

McCammon et al, 1987 p.364

According to Schauben and Frazier (1995) gender seems to be a factor in how rescue workers/counselors choose to cope with secondary traumatic stress/vicarious trauma. In a study on the effect of vicarious traumatic stress on female counselors working with sexual violence survivors, they found the following coping strategies to be most popular among female therapists:

1. **Active coping strategies**, concentrating efforts on doing something about the problem.
2. **Seeking emotional support**, trying to get emotional support from friends and family.
3. **Planning**, make a plan of action.
4. **Seeking instrumental support**, ask someone fro advice on how to deal with situation.
5. **Humor**, laugh about the situation.

Additional strategies that were endorsed were:

1. **Physical health**, including physical exercise, sleeping well, and eating healthy foods.
2. **Spiritually orientated activities** included meditating, being in nature and keeping a journal.
3. **Leisure activities** included listening to music, movies, gardening, and reading.

The least endorsed strategies were:

- Substance abuse
- Denial
- Disengagement / disassociation

All the popular coping strategies were correlated with a significant lower level of distress. On the contrary the least popular strategies all were either unrelated to symptomatology or aggravated the problem.

Sawyer (2001) summarized the issue of self-care by stating that as self-care activities increased symptoms of secondary stress decrease. As self-awareness increased, symptoms of secondary traumatic stress decreased.

2.5 Treatment Programs

2.5.1 Accelerated Recovery Program (ARP) Model

2.5.1.1 Introduction

The Accelerated Recovery Program (ARP) was developed by Gentry, Baranowsky and Dunning (2003) under the direction of Figley for the treatment and prevention of compassion fatigue for a wide variety of professionals. Its aim was to provide individuals with the necessary materials to develop resilience and prevention skills from compassion fatigue. The original model consists of five sessions (later abbreviated into both a three-session and one-day group workshop).

Treatment sessions are standardized and aim to cover the following program goals:

- Symptom identification
- Recognize compassion fatigue triggers
- Identify and utilize resources
- Review personal and professional history to the present day
- Master arousal reduction methods
- Learn grounding and containment skills
- Contract for life enrichment

- Overcome obstacles to effectiveness
- Initiate conflict resolution
- Implement supportive aftercare plan

(Gentry, Baranowsky and Dunning, 2003)

2.5.1.2 ARP Components

1. **Therapeutic Alliance:** This is vital principle of the program that each person who concluded the program will be treated with respect and empathy.

2. **Assessment**

   a) **Quantitive:** The ARP makes use of a compassion fatigue assessment profile, expanded by Stamm (2003) to be the compassion fatigue and satisfaction questionnaire. The package allows one to judge various aspects of compassion fatigue, silencing, primary trauma exposure, emotional disturbance and stressors that may impact on the rescue member's functioning.

   b) **Qualitative:** A participant interview that acknowledges the importance of depathologised, mutual, strength-based approaches with participants.

3. **Anxiety Management:** Each participant is exposed to a variety of anxiety reduction tools to help the individual with the management of stress and reducing negative arousal.

4. **Narrative:** Story telling and the healing quality of personal self-awareness aids in rebuilding professional and personal life quality.

5. **Exposure/Resolution of Secondary Traumatic Stress:** Utilizing exposure techniques in the treatment of anxiety disorders and PTSD is well known. Accordingly it is used in the treatment of compassion fatigue as designed by Wolpe (1969), *The Practice of Behavior Therapy*.

6. **Cognitive Restructuring (Self-care and Integration):** Disputing irrational cognitions help to shift/neutralize automatic thoughts and beliefs that may potentially install negative world views.

7. **Pathways – Self-directed Resiliency and Aftercare Plan:** The PATHWAYS is an integral part of the ARP and comprises an aftercare element that strengthens the participant with a sense of personal commitment to wellness and responsibility.

2.5.1.3 Pathways – Aftercare Resiliency Model

The PATHWAYS program represents the aftercare/ primary prevention component of the ARP model. It compromises of five sections which attempts to enhance skills development and act as a barrier and means of stress tenacity.

Gentry et al (2003) identify five areas which are active involved in the advancement of wellbeing:

1. **Resiliency Skills – Non-anxious Presence and Self-validated Care giving:** The ARP model proposes that professionals who are able to develop and maintain the vital abilities of "non-anxious presence" and "self-validated care giving" will experience a greater than before sense of resiliency to compassion fatigue.
2. **Self-management and Self-care:** Participants of the program are asked to identify what leads them to feel overwhelmed in their occupational of personal lives? What self-protective boundaries need to be implemented or re-enforced? What self-care or self-soothing skills need to be developed, implemented or reinstated or reorganized?
3. **Connection with Others:** Isolation and self-constraint often contributes to compassion fatigue symptoms. Breaking the former cycle can ameliorate the problems associated with compassion fatigue. Participants are asked to face up to and develop neglected means of support, nurturance and enrichment.
4. **Skills Acquisition:** Continuous professional skills development acts as a buffer to compassion fatigue. A lack of professional training and supervision can contribute to feelings of inadequacy and poor self-esteem.

5. **Conflict Resolution:**

- *Internal*: Professionals often know what the necessary coping skills are that would make them cope better with their occupational risks, yet they seldom implement them. Internal conflict may arise, which in tern can cause an energy drain of valuable resources away from issues that are current to personal historical issues.
- *External- Resolution of Primary Traumatic Stress*: Many professional rescue workers have experienced primary traumatic episodes in their personal lives. The former symptomatology may be retriggered through their occupational hazards. It is therefore critical that past traumatic episodes need to be resolved successfully.

As discussed the ARP-model proposes a comprehensive treatment plan for STSD/compassion fatigue. However the lack of quantative data and the interchangeability of a program from individual to group approaches beg the question of scientific validity.

2.5.2 National Institute of Mental Health (USA): Basic Guidelines

2.5.2.1 Introduction

Bisson (2003) quoted the National Institute of Mental Health's published consensus of 2002 regarding aftercare of mass violence as suggesting:

- That it is sensible to expect normal recovery in the immediate post-incident phase
- That participation in early intervention should be voluntary

- That follow-up should be offered to individuals at high risk of developing adjustment difficulties such as those with clinically significant symptoms stemming from the trauma, bereaved individuals, individuals with physical injuries, those with pre-experiencing psychiatric disorder, and those with a particular intense exposure to the traumatic event.

2.5.2.2 Basic Guidelines

Myers and Wee (p.201, 2003) compiled a list of recommendations from the Institute of Mental Health (USA) on the management of stress while working on a disaster operation.

They are divided into 19 steps as follow:

1. *"Request a briefing at the beginning of each shift* to update yourself and your coworkers on the status of things since your last shift. This can help you be more prepared for what you may be encountering during your shift.
2. *Develop a buddy system with a coworker.* Agree to keep an eye on each other's functioning, fatigue level, and stress symptoms. Tell a buddy how to know when you are getting stressed. Make a pact with them to take a break when they suggest it, if the situation allows.
3. *Encourage and support coworkers.* Listen to each others feelings. Don't take anger too personally. Hold criticisms unless essential. Praise each other regarding you work performance.
4. *Try to get some activity and exercise.* Simple use the stairs in stead of the elevator. Gently stretch out muscles that have become tense.
5. *Eat regularly.* If you are not hungry, eat frequently in small quantities. Try to avoid excessive sugar, fats, and caffeine. Drink plenty of liquids.
6. *Use humor to break the tension and provide relief.* Use humor with care. People are highly suggestible in disaster situations, and survivors and coworkers can take things personally and be hurt if they feel they are the brunt of "disaster humor".

7. *Use positive self-talk,* such as "I'm doing fine" and "I am using the skills I've been rained to use".
8. *Take deep breaths, hold them and then blow out forcefully.*
9. *Take breaks if your effectiveness is diminished,* or if asked to do so by your supervisor. At a minimum, take a break every four hours.
10. *Use a clipboard or notebook to jot things down.* This will help for the memory problems that are common in stressful situations.
11. *Try to keep noise to a minimum in the worksite.*
12. *Try to avoid unnecessarily interrupting coworkers* when they are in the middle of a task.
13. *Let yourself defuse at the end of each shift* by taking a few minutes with coworkers to talk about your thoughts and feeling about the day.
14. *When you are off duty, enjoy some recreation that takes your mind off the disaster.* Draw on supports that nurture you. These include friends, meditation, reading and religion.
15. *Pamper yourself during time off.* Treat yourself to a special meal, get a massage, or take along bath.
16. *If needed, give yourself permission to spend time alone after work.* However do not totally withdraw fro social interaction.
17. *Get adequate sleep.* Learn relaxation techniques that can help you fall asleep.
18. *On long disaster assignments, attend periodic debriefing or worker support groups* to talk about the emotional impact on you and on coworkers. Use stress management programs if they are available. If such programs are not offered, try to organize them.
19. *On disaster assignments away from home remember the following:*
    - Try to make your living accommodations as personal, comfortable, and homely as possible. Unpack bags and put out pictures of loved ones.
    - Bring familiar foods and snacks from home that may not be available on your disaster assignment.
    - Make new friends. Let off steam with coworkers.
    - Find local recreation opportunities and make use of them.

- Remember things that are relaxing at home and try to do them now: for
  example take a hot bath, read a good book, or go for a run.
- Stay in touch with people at home. Write or call often. Send pictures. Have
  a family visit if possible.
- Avoid excessive use of alcohol or caffeine.
- Keep a journal."

In conjunction with the former suggestions the National Institute of Mental Health
(USA) recommend that rescue workers be debriefed after a disaster operation,
especially long-term assignments. The purpose of the formal debriefing is to
address the emotional and psychological impact that the disaster assignment has
had on the rescue workers. Myers & Wee (2003) highlight the importance of
empathy, understanding, and peer support generated when the intervention is
performed for a group of rescue workers.

Although most of the suggestions may be viewed as good old fashion common
sense, it is not clear if the National Institute of Mental Health propose these former
guidelines because they have been proven to work (no research data is supplied
to substantiate this) or because they think it may work.

2.5.3 Single Session Early Psychological Interventions

2.5.3.1 Introduction

Single session psychological debriefings have been used with trauma survivors,
emergency care workers, and provides of psychological care. The focus of the
intervention is on present reactions of those involved in trauma instead of personal
historical experiences that may shape an individual's reactions. Psychiatric
labeling is avoided and the emphasis is on normalization. Participants are assured
that they are normal for experiencing the symptoms they do due to an

extraordinary/abnormal that they had experienced, whether it is directly or indirectly (Mitchell, 1983).

2.5.3.2 Critical Incident Stress Management

Critical incident stress debriefing was first formally described by Mitchell in 1983. He proposed a program for an individual or group intervention for ambulance personnel following exposure to traumatic situations in their work (Burns & Harm, 1993; Bisson, 2003). It is designed as a semi-structured intervention with the aim of reducing initial distress and preventing the development of delayed pathology such as PTSD or Secondary Traumatic Stress Disorder, in response to critical incidents. The program is designed to promote emotional processing through the ventilation and normalization of symptom responses and improving resilience for future incidents. Furthermore the program attempts to identify individuals who are vulnerable to complications and who may benefit from more in-depth treatment.

Initially Mitchel (1983) proposed that a follow-up session be scheduled weeks or months later to deal with unresolved issues if necessary. More recently (Mitchell and Everly, 1995) it has been suggested by him that debriefings should be considered as one component of a comprehensive, systematic, multi-component approach (Critical incident Stress Management) to the management of traumatic stresses and that it should not be used in isolation.

Critical incident stress debriefing had initially been described as consisting of six parts (Mitchell, 1983).

1. **The introductory phase:** Participants are introduced to the debriefing team. The therapists discuss expectations and guidelines. The purpose of the program is an opportunity to discuss what happened, a place to learn about common reactions, and time to hear about coping strategies. Group rules, including confidentiality is discussed. Active participation is voluntary.

2. **The fact phase:** Normal reactions to a traumatic event are presented by the facilitator. Participants are then asked for a factual description of exactly what happened by asking them to describe their experience incorporating all sensory modalities (i.e. what had they seen, heard, smelled etc.).

3. **The feeling phase:** The facilitator presents the normal emotional reactions that result from the critical incident. This is accomplished through discussion and presentation of post-trauma stress reactions. Participants are then encouraged to share their feelings be it positive or negative (e.g. fears, anxieties, guilt, anger).

4. **The symptom phase:** This phase encourages participants to discuss various trauma related symptoms they experienced during the traumatic event or subsequently.

5. **The teaching phase:** This part flows from the symptom phase and promotes the discussion of typical symptoms in an attempt to normalize them as a natural stress response.

6. **The reentry phase:** In this phase the facilitator clarifies issues, and gives the opportunity for questions. They discuss the need for direction or specific activity after debriefing. They provide summary comments and ends with closure.

2.5.3.3 Dyregov-model

A similar psychological debriefing model had been developed by Dyregov (1989). It consists of a seven-stage semi-structured intervention adhering closely to Mitchell's model of critical incident stress debriefing. It emphasized the detailed consideration of experiences and emotions at the time of the critical incident as well as afterwards. This he views as a key component in the therapeutic process. Group factors are also considered to play a crucial role in the process.

2.5.3.4 Raphael- model

Raphael (1986) created a psychological debriefing model that is less structured than both the models designed by Mitchell and Dyregov. It however shares many common factors, such as the fact that it was designed as a group intervention for secondary trauma victims rather that survivors of primary traumatic stress. It is recommend by her that particular topics would be useful during the debriefing process.

Some of these are personally experienced disaster stressors such as:

- Personal encounters with death
- Survivor conflict
- Loss and displacement
- Feelings, both positive and negative
- The victims that were rescued and their problems
- The special nature of disaster work
- Any other personal experiences

No track record of efficacy of any of these models has been published. All previous claims of success have also been nullified (Bisson, 2003).

2.5.4 Multiple stressor debriefing model

This model was designed for the use of the American Red Cross personnel (Armstrong, O'Callahan and Marmar, 1991). The model contains elements of the former mentioned trauma debriefing models. The major distinguishing component is that it focuses for the first time on strategies adopted by individuals before the trauma to deal with stressful situations. It is proposed by the program that call-up of similar coping strategies is likely to be of therapeutic value after a traumatic incident (both primary and secondary).

Participants are encouraged to discuss any large number of incidents that were experienced in the weeks or months of their disaster work. In this model questions are framed to encourage discussion of any of a large number of incidents that were challenging or difficult. With participants discussing the events themselves as well as the thoughts, feelings, stress reactions, and coping approaches associated with the events (Myers and Wee, 2003).

The former mentioned debriefing methods are widely being used with individuals as opposed to groups. This has led to criticism by Dyregov (1998) that individual sessions have compromised the therapeutic group factors which are inevitable lost. In any event both approaches have yet to report any scientific data as proof of its efficacy.

2.5.5 Constructivist Self Development Theory as treatment model for Vicarious Traumatization

2.5.5.1 Introduction

Saakvitne and Pearlman (1992) developed a treatment program for vicarious traumatization, based on the constructivist self development al theory developed by Pearlman and McCann (1990); refer to chapter 2.2.

Their introductory comments state that in order to transform vicarious traumatization you need to love your work or some important aspect of it, depicted by Stamm (2003) as compassion satisfaction. It has to be more than a job. Being as difficult and personally demanding as it is, the work has to be done with some personal meaning or conviction. Although vicarious traumatization can obscure this meaning, it is possible to regain it through restoring our lost energy by using the following strategies. If the sense of purpose or meaning is not restored the authors recommend changing careers!

2.5.5.2 Strategies to address the stress of vicarious traumatizaton

Self-care strategies aimed at addressing the stress of vicarious traumatizaton fall into three categories:

1. **Self-care**: includes balance, limits, healthy habits and connection with others.
2. **Self nurturing**: includes gentleness, a focus on pleasure and comfort, relaxation and play.
3. **Escape**: include activities that allow you to forget about work, to engage in fantasy, and to get away from painful memories and feelings.

2.5.5.3 Transforming the loss of meaning by vicarious traumatizaton

The strategies proposed by the Saakvitne and Pearlman (1992) are aimed at allowing the participants to transform vicarious traumatization through infusing meaning into their lives. The strategies challenge the despair, nihilism, and cynicism that result from this condition.

They fall into four categories:

1. **Creating meaning:** the making or discovery of meaning is the antithesis to the erosion or negation of meaning that results from vicarious traumatization.

2. **Infuse a current activity with meaning:** as one has the ability to discover meaning/significance in already familiar activities by consciously infusing them with meaning, whether they are hobbies, playing with one's children, reading philosophy, or civic commitments. Exercise can be transformed from a reluctant trip to the gym to a cherished walk in the woods, where it could include reflection upon the beauty of nature. This kind of mindful, intentional awareness helps one to transform vicarious traumatizaton by reconnecting one with the transient aspects of one's experience, thereby restoring one's spiritual experience.

3. **Challenging negative beliefs and assumptions:** by actively disputing (CBT) or allowing experiences to challenge negative irrational beliefs or cynicism, one would be reclaiming meaning and transforming vicarious traumatization.

4. **Participation in community building activities:** engaging in community activities, whether it is on a small or large scale enables one to reclaim a connection. Cooperating in achieving a common goal or the common good offsets the psychic and spiritual isolation of vicarious traumatization.

2.5.5.4 Awareness, Balance, and Connection

According to Saakvitne and Pearlman (1992) three central aspects of vicarious traumatization interventions are: awareness, balance, and connection.

- **Awareness** reflects on one's attunement to one's needs, limits, emotions, and resources. This awareness of one's inner state and disequilibrium creates the possibility for responsiveness and self-care. Full awareness requires attention to all aspects of one's experience, including dreams, imagination, associations, emotions, bodily sensations, and conscious and preconscious material. An awareness demands time and quiet for reflection.

- **Balance** both within one and life activities are crucial. It provides stability to help one keep one's priorities straight. Balancing work, play and rest activities are essential. It helps us to attend to all aspects of ourselves and thus be more integrated, complete persons.

- **Connection** with others, to us, and to something larger than ourselves provide an antidote to the isolation that is a hallmark of vicarious traumatization. Inner connection allows us greater awareness of our needs, experience and perception. Connection to others, personally and professionally, is critical for trauma workers. If one actively did not stay connected to a larger more complex world, one can get lost in a persecutory maize. The connection with something larger provides an internal anchor for the rescue worker's experience. It breaks the silence of unacknowledged pain and increases validation and hope.

These aspects of self-care ought to be implemented in all the realms of one live, be it professional, organizational or personal. The theory may seem impressive and claim broad strokes of success, yet no data has ever been supplied to substantiate the claims of efficacy.

2.6 Discussion

The management programs of secondary traumatic stress, vicarious traumatization, and compassion fatigue can be seen as being very ambitious and inspiring to the therapist or the client hoping to alleviate the symptoms and ensure a better quality of life. There however certain problems that would need to be taken into consideration.

The ARP-model offers in theory a comprehensive approach to the management of compassion fatigue. Of particular interest is the **PATHWAYS** program that attempts to offer aftercare and act as primary prevention. The individual approach proposed is positively correlated with the findings of a subjective experience of secondary trauma, necessitating a specific approach.

The authors state that they were requested to change the format of the program, for logistical and economical reasons, from a comprehensive five session individual program to a more group focused three sessions, or a one-day workshop. It begs the question as to whether the benefit of the original program would remain intact. If not, the altered program makes no meaningful contribution; if it is the case, it queries the reasons behind the original concept. This document proposes the former to be the case.

At the time of publication in 2003 the authors, Gentry, Baranowsky and Dunning (2003, p133), admitted that , despite of the fact that they make use of the Compassion Fatigue and Compassion Satisfaction Questionnaire which generates quantative data, they had: "very little empirical data on the efficacy, utility and/ safety of this approach."

They claim that several brief trauma codes of behavior have shown promise, yet they do not elaborate on what this claim means. They encourage other therapists to join them in utilizing this protocol, but can offer no quantitative data of successful adaptation as one would expect would be generated from the aforementioned questionnaire.

The management of **Vicarious Traumatization** according to the constructivist self developmental theory is a comprehensive model which proposes certain lifestyle strategies for the rescue professional. The primary problem with this management program is that the authors presuppose a level of sophistication in self awareness and a capacity for self-care. This may almost at times seem like preaching to the converted, meaning an action plan for individuals who already are coping.

The individual that would present with the aforementioned condition typically lacks this level of sophistication or self-awareness. Secondly they often are skilled in rescuing victims from disaster situations in a physical sense. Yet they are not instructed in how to increase a level of emotional awareness and self-care, nor would recommendations as such bring the necessary insight. A more in depth and individualized plan is proposed, that would not only focus on general symptoms of distress but rather attempt to identify subjective etiologies which could aid in the customized treatment plans

The recommendations of the **National Institute of Mental Health** provide practical measures that can ensure effective management of the immediate situation. This falls in line with the suggestions by Bryant, Harvey, Dang and Sackville (1998) that the development of a stepped care approach will prove to be the best way forward.

Furthermore it supports the view by Bisson (2003) that early psychological interventions for survivors of trauma or rescue workers may not guarantee successful management or recovery from the critical incident. Bisson proposes the restriction of broad based immediate psychological interventions, while providing early practical support, including issues such as providing:

- Safety
- Food and shelter
- Assistance getting home
- Assistance contacting relatives
- Assistance in allowing time-off work

However very little guidance is offered on the management of more complex syndromes as may be the case with multiple traumatic incidents.

In the case of **Single and multiple sessions debriefing models**, there remains very little evidence in its efficacy in the management of secondary traumatic stress symptoms. Bisson (2003) proposes that these interventions may actually be detrimental as early intervention may medicalise normal distress. It may also increase the expectance of developing pathological symptoms in those who might otherwise not have done so.

According to Bisson (2003) most individuals experience a normal adjustment process to trauma, involving rapid decrease in psychological symptoms and resolution in a few months' time. This may explain the incidents of efficacy that are reported regarding single session debriefing. The question is then raised as to which factors do necessitate the need for psychological intervention, post-trauma.

The proposal is made that phenomenological factors both past and present offer the most realistic model within which the varied responses and accordingly treatment plans to trauma can be conceptualized. To realize this it is proposed that personality factors which represent the individual's reaction and adjustment to life issues both past, present as well as for the future may offer the necessary information for the therapist in customizing a management program for the people in need of more comprehensive assistance with secondary traumatic stress, vicarious traumatization, or compassion fatigue.

CHAPTER THREE

METHODOLOGY

3.1 Introduction

Symptomatic response to a critical incident is a subjective adaptive process that remains unique to any person. It can therefore be deducted that treatment plans for such symptoms necessitate individualised approaches.

The person can best be understood as an organically unified and unsegmented totality. The focus of personology is on customised solution plans based on individual personality profiles to assist the whole being of the person to adapt according to his/her abilities in becoming "whole" again. This must not be seen as a process of homeostasis but rather as a dynamic growth process/spiral towards self-actualisation.

In considering personality traits that protect or predispose individuals to secondary traumatic stress disorder/compassion fatigue, it is possible to address individual responses to critical incidents in an individualised way. This may improve prognosis for recovery and primary prevention.

A review of the international literature reveals certain relationships between:

- Pre-morbid factors and secondary traumatic stress disorder
- Critical incidents, personality styles and psychological adaptation.
- Personality factors prone individuals to experience peri-traumatic dissociation during critical incidents and secondary traumatic stress disorder.

63

- Personality factors prone individuals to negative interpretations/ schemas of recurrent memories and secondary traumatic stress disorder.

These relationships will be the basis on which the proposed research will attempt to elaborate. In personology it is thought that certain personality styles could possibly act as predictors. This is crucial in the identification and recruiting of emergency rescue staff as well as for appropriate therapeutic interventions for staff that present with STSD/compassion fatigue.

3.2 Objectives

Given the above the **objectives** of the study were to:

1. Determine the prevalence of secondary traumatic stress disorder amongst emergency rescue staff in the study group.

2. Determine the personality traits that predispose South African emergency rescue workers to negative interpretations of recurrent memories and secondary traumatic stress disorder.

3. Determine the psychological adaptation that specific personality styles dictate in times of critical incidents.

4. Make recommendations regarding a personological treatment programme, both primary and secondary in dealing with secondary traumatic stress disorder amongst emergency rescue workers.
5. To implement and assess the efficacy of the Action Centred Personological Treatment Plan.

3.3   Hypothesis

The theoretical basis and gaps in the literature were used as a point of departure in formulating as hypothesis. For the purpose of this study the following hypothesis was generated and tested.

- **An Action Centred Personological Treatment Plan will significantly reduce symptoms of secondary traumatic stress disorder/ compassion fatigue, in the experimental group from pre to post-testing, as well as show significantly fewer symptoms than the control group at post-testing.**

- **An Action Centred Personological Treatment Plan will significantly reduce symptoms of burnout, in the experimental group from pre to post-testing, as well as show significantly fewer symptoms than the control group at post-testing.**

- **An Action Centred Personological Treatment Program will not significantly affect the condition of compassion satisfaction in a negative way, in the experimental group from pre- to post-testing, as well as score significantly higher than the control group at post-testing.**

3.4 Method

3.4.1 Introduction

Research designs can be evaluated according to four criteria:

1. **Spatial control** - the ability to pre-test equality between experimental and control groups.
2. **Temporal control** - the ability to control extraneous factors between pre-tests and post-tests.
3. **Analysis of changes** - the ability of the design to permit analysis of the pre-test and post-test individual scores.
4. **Representativeness** - the ability of the design to be representative in terms of sampling of units and the utilisation of uncontrived or realistic situations that adequately reflect the environment in question (Labovitz & Hagedorn, 1981).

3.4.2 A Quasi-experimental design

In order to determine whether there will be a statistically meaning full reduction in the prevalence of symptoms of secondary traumatic stress disorder (STSD)/compassion fatigue and the co-morbid symptoms of burnout amongst emergency rescue staff who had been instructed in an Action Centred Personological Treatment Plan, a test re- test quasi-experimental analysis with two independent groups was required.

Existing psychometric assessment instruments were utilised to generate data for the experimental analysis. The quantitative data was supported by information gathered from a clinical social history questionnaire. This information was used as part of the discussion of the results as a means to enhance the former descriptive results.

3.4.3 Participants and sampling

In an effort to attain spatial and temporal control a sample population was selected with a cluster sampling method from the greater Gauteng emergency rescue staff. They included paramedics, fire fighters and ambulance staff. The specific municipality had been incorporated into a greater Gauteng metropolis in the past two years. As they were still in transitional phase at the time of the intervention certain circumstantial stress factors were noted from the respondents' remarks.

Among the factors that were mentioned by the respondents the following were the most frequent:

i)   Poor and inconsistent management styles
ii) Shifts of 24 hours and even 72 hours over weekends compared to the other municipality's 12 hour shifts.
iii) Animosity among staff as well as among staff and management.
iv) The reality of affirmative action and its unique challenges with regard to equity vs. competency and experience.

Potential subjects for both the experimental and control group were obtained through drawing personnel files, using random sampling in March 2004. A sample of 17 participants was included in the intervention group and 17 participants were included in a non-intervention group. This was representative of 80% of the total population group of emergency rescue staff in this particular municipality.

By randomly assigning subjects to the two groups, the effects of unknown and known variables were, within probability limits, equally distributed (Labovitz and Hagedorn, 1981). For the purposes of this study, subjects participating in the Action Centred Personological Treatment Plan were referred to as the "experimental group", whereas subjects who did not participate in the former treatment plan were referred to as the "control group".

As South Africa is renowned for its multicultural composition, there are concerns with regard to cross-cultural validity and reliability in the application of "western" psychological tests. These concerns are acknowledged. A quasi-experimental design was proposed where variables will be measured on a pre-test, post-test basis. However every system is unique and dynamic. Therefore the selected experimental- and control groups can be considered to be temporal systems, inclusive of a multi-cultural dimension.

3.5 Measurement Instruments

3.5.1 Personal History Questionnaire

A personal history questionnaire was developed and applied to gather information on the personal-social history of the subjects. It did, *inter alia*, serve to elicit information on:

- Educational qualification
- Age
- Years of service
- Gender
- Ethnicity
- Psychiatric history
- History of exposure to critical incidents

3.5.2 Millon Index of Personality Styles

The Millon Index of Personality Styles (MIPS) is a 180-item; true/false questionnaire designed to measure personality styles of normally functional adults between the ages of 18 and 65+. Most MIPS items require an eighth-grade (or its equivalent) education to complete.

The MIPS consists of 24 scales grouped into 12 pairs. Each pair contains two juxtaposed scales. The MIPS scales are organised into three major areas: Motivating Aims, Cognitive Modes, and Interpersonal Behaviours. In addition to the 12 pairs of content scales, the MIPS-questionnaire contains three validity indicators: Positive Impression, Negative Impression, and Consistency.

Three pairs of Motivating-Aims scales asses the person's orientation toward obtaining reinforcement from the environment. The first pair of scales examines the extent to which he respondent's behaviour is basically motivated by obtaining positive reinforcement or avoiding negative stimulation from the world. The second pair assesses the extent to which the individual's activities reflect a modifying or accommodating approach to the world. The third pair's of scales focuses on the source of reinforcement, assessing to which extent the persons are motivated by themselves or the world.

Four pairs of Cognitive-Modes scales examine styles of information processing. The first two pairs in this area assess information-gathering strategies. The second two pairs assess different styles of processing information once it has been gathered.
Five pairs of Interpersonal-Behaviours scales assess the person's style of relating to others in general incorporating social skills, assertiveness skills and conflict management skills.

Each style represents adaptive patterns that fit certain environments and situations quite well and others less well (Millon, 1994). No norm scores have yet been standardised for the South African population. In the development and standardisation of the MIPS in the United States of America a cross-cultural subject group was utilised. It comprised of 11,3% African American, 7,5% Hispanic, 79,5% White and 1,7% other ethnic groups.

For internal-consistency reliability, median coefficient alphas were generally in the upper 0,70's, and the median split-half reliabilities were typically in the low 0,80's.

Median retest reliabilities were in the middle 0,80's across the various samples examined. Although the constructs measured by the MIPS are not highly one-dimensional or homogeneous, the scales are nonetheless quite dependable, stable and reliable over time (Millon, 1994).

3.5.3 Search and Rescue Society of British Columbia Burnout Questionnaire

The Burnout Questionnaire of the Search and Rescue Society of British Columbia is a 15-item questionnaire measuring a respondent's symptomatic status with regard to burnout and compassion fatigue. The questionnaire is scored on a Likert scale from 1 to 5. It questions individuals on whether there have been any negative changes in the respondents over the past 6 months. Subjects will place themselves on an attitude continuum for each statement- running from 1 for no or very little change to 5 for a great deal of change.

The results from this questionnaire were compared with scores obtained from the MIPS and Compassion Fatigue and Satisfaction Questionnaire to explore any meaningful correlations.

3.5.4 Compassion Satisfaction and Fatigue Test

The Compassion Satisfaction and Fatigue Test (CSF-test) was the combined effort of Figley's (1995) Compassion Fatigue Test Revised (CSFT-R) and Stamm's (2003) Compassion Satisfaction component. It comprises of 66-item questionnaire measuring the respondent's symptomatic status on the following scales:

- Compassion Fatigue
- Compassion satisfaction
- Burnout

The questionnaire is scored on a Likert scale from 0 for never to 5 for very often. It attempted to identify both the costs of caring as well as the positive payments of doing caring work for people in distress.

The combined sample group consisted of 374 individuals from among others South Africa, Canada and the United States of America. The overall alpha median scores for the scales ranged from .87 for STSD/compassion fatigue and compassion satisfaction, and .90 for burnout (Stamm, 2003). Although the results are preliminary, they are consistent with the findings of Figley and Stamm (1996), who reported reliabilities of .85 to .94 on a sample of 142 psychotherapy therapists.

3.6 Treatment intervention procedure

Both groups were pre-tested in separate group sessions for the prevalence of secondary traumatic stress disorder/compassion fatigue, burnout and general emotional adjustment. There after the experimental group were treated on an individual basis with the Action Centred Personological Treatment Plan.

The intervention was conducted in the following manner:

1. A group interview for orientation and comprehensive assessment of personality structure (psychometric testing). Experimental and control groups were consulted separately.

2. **Ninety minute individual feedback / action planning session with each subject in the experimental group.** The session focused on relaying feedback to the client on his/her scores on the various tests re STSD/compassion fatigue, burnout and compassion satisfaction. Personality styles from the MIPS were identified that may aggravate their current emotional condition regarding the former scores. Specific CBT exercises and general life skills were customised to the individual's needs and abilities and

71

compiled into an action plan incorporating specific homework tasks such as: thought stopping exercises (Wolpe, 1958), emotional journals, daily planners, progressive relaxation and breathing techniques, creative problem solving and general stress management techniques.

3. Fourteen days for trial implementation.

4. **First individual follow-up session with subjects in the experimental group (Approximately 60 minutes).** Subjects reported back on their personal progress on the former CBT action plan. Further personality styles/needs were identified that may complicate recovery and general functioning. Specific focus was generally on negative self beliefs/life scripts, as identified in MIPS that predispose the subject to susceptibility for STSD/compassion fatigue and burnout. More CBT exercises (disputing negative self beliefs through specific journal entries incorporating aspects of self-confession, self-apology, self-forgiveness and gratitude) and further life skills were formulated to the individual's specific needs in their next homework assignment.

5. Thirty day period for implementation

6. **Second individual follow-up session with subjects in the experimental group (Approximately 60 minutes).** Subjects reported back on progress. Any outstanding matters (if applicable) regarding STSD/compassion fatigue and burnout were highlighted and addressed with additional CBT action plans for future use.

The reasons for an individual approach versus a group approach were:

- To promote ethics in the experimental study.
- To promote the principle of individualised treatment plans to staff needs.
- To limit the risk of personal embarrassment and inhibition.
- To promote staff members rights to privacy and anonymity.
- To limit staff members concerns about group esteem if colleagues were to know certain personal details, which may lead to false positive self-representations of their personal situation.

After the intervention had been implemented on the experimental group over a period of three months both the experimental group and control group were re-tested individually for the prevalence of STSD/compassion fatigue, burnout, compassion fatigue and general emotional adjustment.

Of noted interest was that the only reason that were mentioned as a critical incident catalyst to STSD/compassion fatigue was witnessing the death or serious injury to children, especially among rescue workers who were parents themselves.

3.7   Data analysis

The chief objective of the data analysis was to determine whether there is statistically a significant difference in the prevalence of symptoms of secondary traumatic stress disorder/compassion fatigue, burnout and compassion satisfaction (the dependant variables) in the subjects of the experimental group versus the control group before and after the Action Centred Personological Treatment Programme (the independent or treatment variable) had been implemented on the experimental group.

The data was analysed for intra- and inter group correlations using the t-distribution for two unpaired samples using estimated variances. The assumption is that the design consists of two samples chosen randomly from normal distributions. Of further note is that the assumption is made that both populations had the same variance.

A Wilcoxon Signed Ranks Test was used to determine the significance of difference between the pre- and post-test scores of the experimental group and control group on the dependant variables as discussed. As the population values are large ($N > 16$) a normal approximation for the null hypothesis distribution of $T+$ was used (Clarke and Cooke, 2004).

3.8. Ethical considerations

Permission had been obtained from the Executive Director Human Resources from the specific metropolitan council. Subjects participated on a voluntary basis. All personal information was treated confidential.

The control group was not treated with the Action Centred Personological Treatment Programme. The metropolitan council will be given the option to implement this programme on all the remaining emergency rescue staff.

3.9 Concluding remarks

In this chapter the research hypotheses and objectives were formulated and a discussion of the methodology was presented. Certain qualititive data regarding circumstantial stresses and catalysts to STSD/compassion fatigue were reported. A report of the statistical results follows in the next chapter.

CHAPTER FOUR

RESULTS

4.1 Introduction

Studies on the impact and containment of secondary traumatic stress on South African emergency rescue workers are scarce, despite being an urgent humanitarian crisis for the people concerned. It is therefore necessary to determine the factors that contribute to the phenomena and identify effective strategies of intervention. Clinical personology, incorporating the principles of cognitive behavioral therapy has been offered as a possible model to address the condition successfully. The usage of sound methodological procedures plays a significant role in the investigation of relevant interventions programs as it allows for replication and broader application.

This chapter will provide a statistical analysis of the impact of an individualized action centered personological intervention program, in the treatment of secondary traumatic stress disorder and burnout in emergency rescue staff.

4.2 Hypotheses

1. **An Action Centred Personological Treatment Plan will significantly reduce symptoms of secondary traumatic stress disorder/ compassion fatigue, in the experimental group from pre- to post-testing, as well as show significantly fewer symptoms than the control group at post-testing.**

2. An Action Centred Personological Treatment Plan will significantly reduce symptoms of burnout, in the experimental group from pre- to post-testing, as well as show significantly fewer symptoms than the control group at post-testing.

3. An Action Centred Personological Treatment Plan will not significantly affect the condition of compassion satisfaction in a negative way, in the experimental group from pre- to post-testing, as well as score significantly higher than the control group at post-testing.

In order to test these hypotheses raw data was used collected from the British Columbia Life Style Quiz on Burnout, Compassion Fatigue and Satisfaction Questionnaire, to determine whether symptoms of burnout and compassion fatigue/ secondary traumatic stress disorder were present. The data of the Millon Inventory of Personality Styles were used to measure any co-morbid symptoms of depression and anxiety that would typically be associated with secondary traumatic stress. The data was also utilised to customise the solution feedback to the client. These tests are discussed in detail in Chapter 3.

4.3 Experimental Design

4.3.1 Quantitive Analysis

The data will be evaluated by firstly comparing the pre-and post-test levels of the dependant variables for the experimental group, between the group members to determine whether the programme made any significant difference in the prevalence of symptoms discussed, following the intervention program.

The results of the control group will be evaluated by comparing their pre-and post-test scores internally, to determine any significant difference in the prevalence of the symptoms discussed **without receiving the intervention program.**

The results of the pre-and post-test scores of the experimental group will then be compared with the pre-and post-test scores of the control group to determine if there were any significant differences in the inter group results both before the intervention was implemented as well as thereafter.

The dependant variables concerned will be the results of the British Columbia Lifestyle Quiz, the Compassion Fatigue and Satisfaction Questionnaire and the following scores of the personality styles generated by the Millon Inventory of Personality Styles:

- Enhancing
- Preserving
- Yielding
- Complaining

Not all the personality style scores of the latter were used in measuring change after the therapeutic intervention as the bulk of the scores rather serve a heuristic function in customising the therapeutic plan for the individual's needs and abilities. Accordingly it would be more meaningful to interpret to interpret the MIPS results on an individual (intra-personal) basis to gain its full meaning. The full descriptive statistical report can be found in Adendum 1 and 2.

4.3.1.1 Significance of differences between the pre- and post- test mean scores of the experimental group on CFSQ-Secondary Traumatic Stress Disorder / Compassion Fatigue

The critical values for compassion fatigue as set out by Figley (1995) are as follow:

0-26 :   Extremely low risk of compassion fatigue
27-30:   Low risk of compassion fatigue
31-35:   Moderate risk of compassion fatigue
36-40:   High risk of compassion fatigue
41 +:   Extremely high risk of compassion fatigue

The mean values for the experimental group before and after the therapeutic intervention are as follow:

Table 4.1   Comparison of differences between the pre- and post-test mean scores of the experimental group on Secondary Traumatic Stress Disorder/ Compassion Fatigue

	N	Minimum	Maximum	Mean	Std. Deviation
Pre CFSQ Compassion Fatigue	17	29.0	74.0	51.529	14.2921
Post CFSQ Compassion Fatigue	17	8.0	56.0	35.353	12.3235
CF	17	2.00	5.00	4.4706	.87447
PCF	17	1.00	5.00	3.2941	1.64942

The differences between the pre- and post-test mean scores of the experimental group on Secondary Traumatic Stress Disorder/ Compassion Fatigue seem to be significant. The averages of the pre-test scores (51.5) for the experiment al group match that of the category of extreme high risk of compassion fatigue.

The averages of the post-test scores (35.3) for the experimental group match the category of moderate risk of compassion fatigue (see Figure 4.1)

Figure 4.1 **Comparison of differences between the pre- and post-test mean scores of the experimental group on Secondary Traumatic Stress Disorder/ Compassion Fatigue**

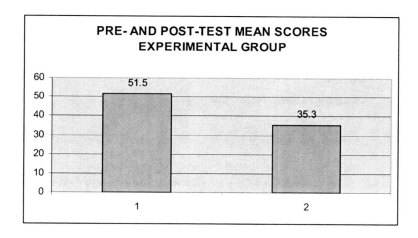

A Wilcoxon Signed Ranks Test which was used to determine the significance of difference between experimental variable on compassion fatigue before the intervention and after the intervention revealed that there is a significant difference between the pre-test scores and post-test scores of the experimental group (see table 4.2).

Table 4.2   Wilcoxon Signed Ranks Test for significance of differences between the pre- and post-test mean scores of the experimental group on Secondary Traumatic Stress Disorder/ Compassion Fatigue

		N	Mean Rank	Sum of Ranks	Post CF – Pre CF
Post CF – Pre CF	Negative Ranks	15	8.87	133.00	
	Positive Ranks	1	3.00	3.00	
	Ties	1			
	Total	17			Z= -3.364
	Asymp. Sig. (2-tailed)				.001

4.3.1.2 Significance of differences between the pre- and post- test mean scores of the control group on CFSQ- Secondary Traumatic Stress Disorder / Compassion Fatigue

The mean values for the control group pre-and post-test are as follow:

Table 4.3   Comparison of differences between the pre- and post-test mean scores of the control group on Secondary Traumatic Stress Disorder/ Compassion Fatigue

	N	Minimum	Maximum	Mean	Std. Deviation
PreCF	17	6.0	85.0	45.471	17.0518
PostCF	17	9.0	85.0	51.294	19.6366
CF	17	1.00	5.00	4.4118	1.12132
PCF	17	1.00	5.00	4.2941	1.15999

The differences between the pre- and post-test mean scores of the control group on Secondary Traumatic Stress Disorder/ Compassion Fatigue seem to be insignificant. The averages of the pre-test scores (45.5) for the experiment al group match that of the category of extreme high risk of compassion fatigue.

The averages of the post-test scores (51.3) for the control group remain in the category of extreme high risk of compassion fatigue (see Figure 4.2)

Figure 4.2   Comparison of differences between the pre- and post-test mean scores of the control group on Secondary Traumatic Stress Disorder/ Compassion Fatigue

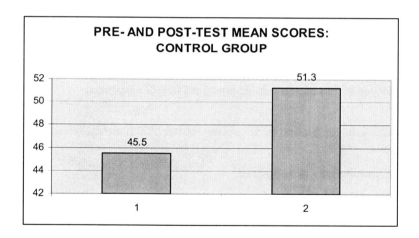

A Wilcoxon Signed Ranks Test which was used to determine the significance of difference between experimental variable on compassion fatigue before the intervention and after the intervention revealed that there is an insignificant difference between the pre-test scores and post-test scores of the control group (see table 4.4).

Table 4.4   Wilcoxon Signed Ranks Test for significance of differences between the pre- and post-test mean scores of the control group on Secondary Traumatic Stress Disorder/ Compassion Fatigue

		N	Mean Rank	Sum of Ranks	Post CF – Pre CF
Post CF – Pre CF	Negative Ranks	6	9.08	54.50	
	Positive Ranks	11	8.95	98.50	
	Ties	0			
	Total	17			Z= -1.042
	Asymp. Sig. (2-tailed)				.297

4.3.1.3 Significance of differences between the pre- and post- test mean scores of the experimental group on CFSQ – Burnout

The critical values for burnout as set out by Stamm (2003) are as follow:

0-36 :   Extremely low risk of burnout
37-50:   Moderate risk of burnout
51-75:   High risk of burnout
76-85:   Extremely high risk of burnout

The mean values for the experimental group before and after the therapeutic intervention are as follow:

Table 4.5 Comparison of differences between the pre- and post-test mean scores of the experimental group on CFSQ- Burnout

	N	Minimum	Maximum	Mean	Std. Deviation
Pre BO	17	19.0	55.0	42.353	8.9229
Post BO	17	8.0	49.0	30.647	11.4069
BO	17	1.00	5.00	4.1765	1.13111
PBO	17	1.00	5.00	2.8235	1.55062

The differences between the pre- and post-test mean scores of the experimental group on CFSQ- Burnout seem to be significant. The averages of the pre-test scores (42.4) for the experiment al group match that of the category of moderate risk of CFSQ-burnout. The averages of the post-test scores (30.6) for the experimental group match the category of extremely low risk of CFSQ- burnout (see Figure 4.3)

Figure 4.3 Comparison of differences between the pre- and post-test mean scores of the experimental group on CFSQ- Burnout

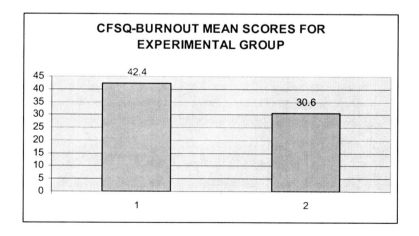

83

A Wilcoxon Signed Ranks Test which was used to determine the significance of difference between experimental variable on CFSQ-Burnout before the intervention and after the intervention revealed that there is a significant difference between the pre-test scores and post-test scores of the experimental group (see table 4.6).

Table 4.6 **Wilcoxon Signed Ranks Test for significance of differences between the pre- and post-test mean scores of the experimental group on CFSQ- Burnout**

Post BO- Pre BO		N	Mean Rank	Sum of Ranks	Post BO- Pre BO
	Negative Ranks	16	9.31	149.00	
	Positive Ranks	1	4.00	4.00	
	Ties	0			
	Total	17			Z= -3.435
	Asymp. Sig. (2-tailed)				.001

4.3.1.4 Significance of differences between the pre- and post- test mean scores of the control group on CFSQ - Burnout

The mean values for the control group pre-and post-test are as follow:

Table 4.7 **Comparison of differences between the pre- and post-test mean scores of the control group on CFSQ- Burnout**

	N	Minimum	Maximum	Mean	Std. Deviation
Pre BO	17	7.0	68.0	41.471	17.1505
Post BO	17	7.0	83.0	41.706	17.8142

The differences between the pre- and post-test mean scores of the control group on CFSQ- Burnout seem to be insignificant. The averages of the pre-test scores (41.4) for the experiment al group match that of the category of moderate risk of burnout. The averages of the post-test scores (41.7) for the control group remain in the category of moderate risk of CFSQ- burnout (see Figure 4.4)

Figure 4.4   Comparison of differences between the pre- and post-test mean scores of the control group on CFSQ- Burnout

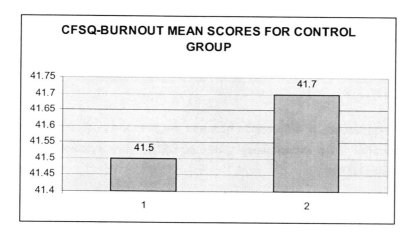

A Wilcoxon Signed Ranks Test which was used to determine the significance of difference between experimental variable on CFSQ-Burnout before the intervention and after the intervention revealed that there is an insignificant difference between the pre-test scores and post-test scores of the control group (see table 4.8).

Table 4.8 **Wilcoxon Signed Ranks Test for significance of differences between the pre- and post-test mean scores of the control group on CFSQ - Burnout**

		N	Mean Rank	Sum of Ranks	Post BO – Pre BO
Post BO – Pre BO	Negative Ranks	8(g)	10.50	84.00	
	Positive Ranks	8(h)	6.50	52.00	
	Ties	1(i)			
	Total	17			Z= -.828
	Asymp. Sig. (2-tailed)				.408

4.3.1.5 Significance of differences between the pre- and post- test mean scores of the experimental group on CFSQ – Compassion Satisfaction

The critical values for compassion satisfaction as set out by Stamm (2003) are as follow:

0-63:   Low potential for compassion satisfaction
64-81:   Modest potential for compassion satisfaction
82-99:   Good potential for compassion satisfaction
100-117:   High potential for compassion satisfaction
118 + :   Extremely high potential for compassion satisfaction

The mean values for the experimental group before and after the therapeutic intervention are as follow:

Table 4.9 Comparison of differences between the pre- and post-test mean scores of the experimental group on CFSQ- Compassion Satisfaction

	N	Minimum	Maximum	Mean	Std. Deviation
Pre CS	17	56.0	117.0	81.588	16.6022
Post CS	17	6.0	119.0	72.235	29.1709

The differences between the pre- and post-test mean scores of the experimental group on CFSQ- Compassion Satisfaction seem to be insignificant. The averages of the pre-test scores (81.6) for the experiment al group match that of the category of modest to good potential for CFSQ-compassion satisfaction. The averages of the post-test scores (72.2) for the experimental group match the category of modest potential for CFSQ- compassion satisfaction (see Figure 4.5).

Figure 4.5 Comparison of differences between the pre- and post-test mean scores of the experimental group on CFSQ- Compassion Satisfaction

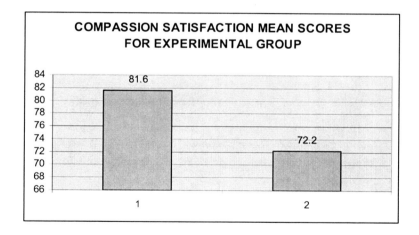

87

A Wilcoxon Signed Ranks Test which was used to determine the significance of difference between experimental variable on CFSQ-Compassion Satisfaction before the intervention and after the intervention revealed that there is an insignificant difference between the pre-test scores and post-test scores of the experimental group (see table 4.10).

Table 4.10 **Wilcoxon Signed Ranks Test for significance of differences between the pre- and post-test mean scores of the experimental group on CFSQ- Compassion Satisfaction**

		N	Mean Rank	Sum of Ranks	Post CS – Pre CS
Post CS- Pre CS	Negative Ranks	9	10.72	96.50	
	Positive Ranks	8	7.06	56.50	
	Ties	0			
	Total	17			Z= -.947
	Asymp. Sig. (2-tailed)				.343

4.3.1.6 Significance of differences between the pre- and post- test mean scores of the control group on CFSQ – Compassion Satisfaction

The mean values for the control group pre-and post-test are as follow:

Table 4.11 **Comparison of differences between the pre- and post-test mean scores of the control group on CFSQ- Compassion Satisfaction**

	N	Minimum	Maximum	Mean	Std. Deviation
Pre CS	17	48.0	123.0	79.176	19.6604
Post CS	17	29.0	111.0	76.706	23.2426

The differences between the pre- and post-test mean scores of the control group on CFSQ- Compassion Satisfaction seem to be insignificant. The averages of the pre-test scores (79.2) for the experimental group match that of the category of modest potential for CFSQ-compassion satisfaction. The averages of the post-test scores (76.7) for the experimental group match the category of modest potential for CFSQ- compassion satisfaction (see Figure 4.6).

Figure 4.6   Comparison of differences between the pre- and post-test mean scores of the control group on CFSQ- Compassion Satisfaction

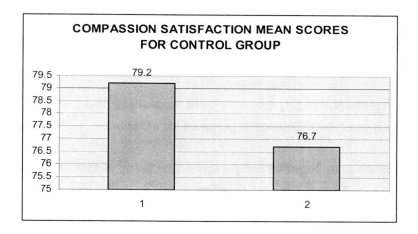

A Wilcoxon Signed Ranks Test which was used to determine the significance of difference between experimental variable on CFSQ-Compassion Satisfaction before the intervention and after the intervention revealed that there is an insignificant difference between the pre-test scores and post-test scores of the control group (see table 4.12).

Table 4.12 Wilcoxon Signed Ranks Test for significance of differences between the pre- and post-test mean scores of the control group on CFSQ-Compassion Satisfaction

		N	Mean Rank	Sum of Ranks	Post CS – Pre CS
Post CS - Pre CS	Negative Ranks	9	10.69	85.50	
	Positive Ranks	8	7.50	67.50	
	Ties	0			
	Total	17			Z= -.426
	Asymp. Sig. (2-tailed)				.670

4.3.1.7 Significance of differences between the pre- and pos- test mean scores of the experimental group on LQ - Burnout

The critical values for burnout as set out by the Search and Rescue Society of British Columbia Burnout Life Style Questionnaire (LQ) are as follow:

0-25 : Extremely low risk of burnout

26-35: Modest risk of burnout

36-50: Significant risk of burnout

51-65: High risk of burnout

65 + : Extremely high risk of burnout

The mean values for the experimental group before and after the therapeutic intervention are as follow:

Table 4.13   Comparison of differences between the pre- and post-test mean scores of the experimental group on LQ- Burnout

	N	Minimum	Maximum	Mean	Std. Deviation
Pre LQ	17	31.0	71.0	43.706	10.0919
Post LQ	17	15.0	52.0	34.529	12.4153
BO	17	1.00	5.00	4.1765	1.13111
PBO	17	1.00	5.00	2.8235	1.55062

The differences between the pre- and post-test mean scores of the experimental group on LQ- Burnout seem to be significant. The averages of the pre-test scores (43.7) for the experiment al group match that of the category of significant risk of LQ-burnout. The averages of the post-test scores (34.6) for the experimental group match the category of modest risk of LQ- burnout (see Figure 4.7)

Figure 4.7   Comparison of differences between the pre- and post-test mean scores of the experimental group on LQ- Burnout

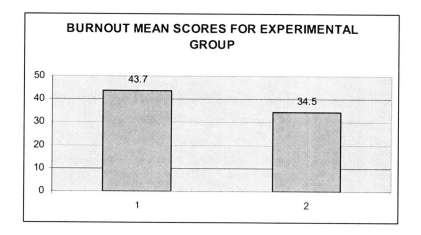

A Wilcoxon Signed Ranks Test which was used to determine the significance of difference between experimental variable on LQ-Burnout before the intervention and after the intervention revealed that there is a significant difference between the pre-test scores and post-test scores of the experimental group (see table 4.14).

Table 4.14   Wilcoxon Signed Ranks Test for significance of differences between the pre- and post-test mean scores of the experimental group on LQ-Burnout

		N	Mean Rank	Sum of Ranks	Post LQ - Pre LQ
Post LQ - Pre LQ	Negative Ranks	13	9.50	123.50	
	Positive Ranks	3	4.17	12.50	
	Ties	1			
	Total	17			Z= -2.87
	Asymp. Sig. (2-tailed)				.004

4.3.1.8 Significance of differences between the pre- and post- rest mean scores of the control group on LQ - Burnout

The mean values for the control group pre-and post-test are as follow:

Table 4.15 Comparison of differences between the pre- and post-test mean scores of the control group on LQ- Burnout

	N	Minimum	Maximum	Mean	Std. Deviation
Pre LQ	17	19.0	70.0	43.824	12.7193
Post LQ	17	17.0	68.0	40.882	12.8932
PLQ	17	1.00	5.00	2.8235	1.07444
LQ	17	1.00	5.00	3.0588	1.02899

The differences between the pre- and post-test mean scores of the control group on LQ- Burnout seem to be insignificant. The averages of the pre-test scores (43.8) for the control group match that of the category of significant risk of LQ-burnout. The averages of the post-test scores (40.8) for the control group match the category of significant risk of LQ- burnout (see Figure 4.8)

Figure 4.8   Comparison of differences between the pre- and post-test mean scores of the control group on LQ- Burnout

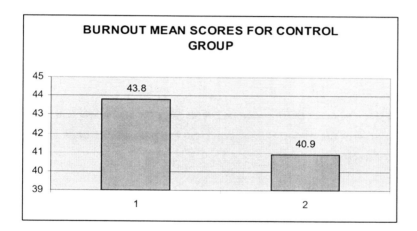

A Wilcoxon Signed Ranks Test which was used to determine the significance of difference between experimental variable on LQ-Burnout before the intervention and after the intervention revealed that there is an insignificant difference between the pre-test scores and post-test scores of the control group (see table 4.16).

Table 4.16   Wilcoxon Signed Ranks Test for significance of differences between the pre- and post-test mean scores of the control group on LQ-Burnout

		N	Mean Rank	Sum of Ranks
Post LQ - Pre LQ	Negative Ranks	12	8.71	104.50
	Positive Ranks	5	9.70	48.50
	Ties	0		
	Total	17		
LQ – PLQ	Negative Ranks	2	5.50	11.00
	Positive Ranks	6	4.17	25.00
	Ties	9		
	Total	17		

4.3.1.9 Significance of differences between the pre- and post- test mean scores of the experimental group on the personality style MIPS: Enhancing

The prevalence scores (PS) on the Millon Inventory of Personality Styles are regarded as being significant for PS values of 50 or higher. PS values that score lower than 50 are regarded as not being a significant personality style of the candidate. For a comprehensive description of the personality style, Enhancing, see chapter 3.

The mean values for the experimental group before and after the therapeutic intervention are as follow:

Table 4.17 Comparison of differences between the pre- and post-test mean scores of the experimental group on MIPS: Enhancing

	N	Minimum	Maximum	Mean	Std. Deviation
Pre Enhan	17	1.0	70.0	43.176	18.9118
Post Enhan	17	13.0	86.0	51.882	23.0540

The differences between the pre- and post-test mean scores of the experimental group on MIPS: Enhancing seem to be significant in terms of the criteria set out by Millon (1994). The pre-test mean scores (43.2) for the experiment al group match that of the category of insignificant prevalence of the personality style, Enhancing. The post-test mean scores (51.9) for the experimental group match the category of significant prevalence of the personality style, Enhancing (see Figure 4.9).

Figure 4.9 Comparison of differences between the pre- and post-test mean scores of the experimental group on MIPS: Enhancing

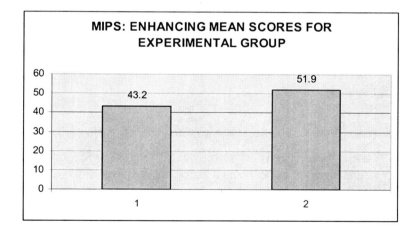

A Wilcoxon Signed Ranks Test which was used to determine the significance of difference between experimental variable on MIPS: Enhancing before the intervention and after the intervention revealed that there is statistically not a significant difference between the pre-test scores and post-test scores of the experimental group (see table 4.18).

Table 4.18   Wilcoxon Signed Ranks Test for significance of differences between the pre- and post-test mean scores of the experimental group on MIPS: Enhancing

		N	Mean Rank	Sum of Ranks	Post Enhan - Pre Enhan
Post Enhan- Pre Enhan	Negative Ranks	5	5.20	26.00	
	Positive Ranks	10	9.40	94.00	
	Ties	2			
	Total	17			Z= -1.932
	Asymp. Sig. (2-tailed)				.053

4.3.1.10 Significance of differences between the pre- and post- test mean scores of the control group on the personality style MIPS: Enhancing

The prevalence scores (PS) on the Millon Inventory of Personality styles are regarded as being significant for PS values of 50 or higher. PS values that score lower than 50 are regarded as not being a significant personality style of the candidate. For a comprehensive description of the personality style, Enhancing, see chapter 3.

The mean values for the control group before and after the therapeutic intervention are as follow:

Table 4.19 Comparison of differences between the pre- and post-test mean scores of the control group on MIPS: Enhancing

	N	Minimum	Maximum	Mean	Std. Deviation
Pre Enhan	17	.0	80.0	42.059	28.6192
Post Enhan	17	.0	86.0	46.471	30.0835

The differences between the pre- and post-test mean scores of the experimental group on MIPS: Enhancing seem to be insignificant in terms of the criteria set out by Millon (1994). The pre-test mean scores (42.1) for the experiment al group match that of the category of insignificant prevalence of the personality style, Enhancing. The post-test mean scores (46.5) for the experimental group match the category of insignificant prevalence of the personality style, Enhancing (see Figure 4.10).

Figure 4.10 Comparison of differences between the pre- and post-test mean scores of the control group on MIPS: Enhancing

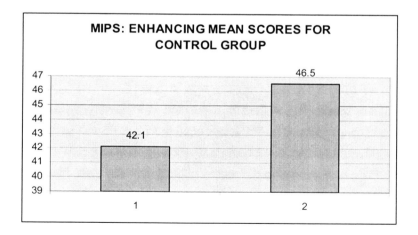

97

A Wilcoxon Signed Ranks Test which was used to determine the significance of difference between control variable on MIPS: Enhancing before the intervention and after the intervention revealed that there is statistically not a significant difference between the pre-test scores and post-test scores of the experimental group (see table 4.20).

Table 4.20   Wilcoxon Signed Ranks Test for significance of differences between the pre- and post-test mean scores of the control group on MIPS: Enhancing

		N	Mean Rank	Sum of Ranks	Post Enhan - Pre Enhan
Post Enhan-Pre Enhan	Negative Ranks	3	8.83	26.50	
	Positive Ranks	10	6.45	64.50	
	Ties	4			
	Total	17			Z= -1.329
	Asymp. Sig. (2-tailed)				.184

4.3.1.11 Significance of differences between the pre- and post test mean scores of the experimental group on the personality style MIPS:Preserving

The prevalence scores (PS) on the Millon Inventory of Personality styles are regarded as being significant for PS values of 50 or higher. PS values that score lower than 50 are regarded as not being a significant personality style of the candidate. For a comprehensive description of the personality style, Preserving, see chapter 3.

The mean values for the experimental group before and after the therapeutic intervention are as follow:

Table 4.21 Comparison of differences between the pre- and post-test mean scores of the experimental group on MIPS: Preserving

	N	Minimum	Maximum	Mean	Std. Deviation
Pre Preserv	17	22.0	100.0	53.706	22.0391
Post Preserv	17	9.0	95.0	44.765	22.4096

The differences between the pre- and post-test mean scores of the experimental group on MIPS: Preserving seem to be significant in terms of the criteria set out by Millon (1994). The pre-test mean scores (53.7) for the experiment al group match that of the category of significant prevalence of the personality style, Preserving. The post-test mean scores (44.8) for the experimental group match the category of insignificant prevalence of the personality style, Preserving (see Figure 4.9).

Figure 4.11 Comparison of differences between the pre- and post-test mean scores of the experimental group on MIPS: Preserving

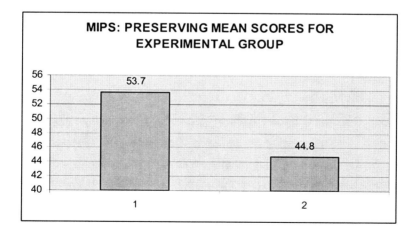

99

A Wilcoxon Signed Ranks Test which was used to determine the significance of difference between experimental variable on MIPS: Preserving before the intervention and after the intervention revealed that there is statistically not a significant difference between the pre-test scores and post-test scores of the experimental group (see table 4.20).

Table 4.22   Wilcoxon Signed Ranks Test for significance of differences between the pre- and post-test mean scores of the experimental group on MIPS: Preserving

		N	Mean Rank	Sum of Ranks	Post Preserv - Pre Preserv
Post Preserv - Pre Preserv	Negative Ranks	13	9.00	117.00	
	Positive Ranks	4	9.00	36.00	
	Ties	0			
	Total	17			Z= -1.918
	Asymp. Sig. (2-tailed)				.055

4.3.1.12 Significance of the differences between the pre- and post- test mean scores of the control group on the personality style MIPS:Preserving

The prevalence scores (PS) on the Millon Inventory of Personality styles are regarded as being significant for PS values of 50 or higher. PS values that score lower than 50 are regarded as not being a significant personality style of the candidate. For a comprehensive description of the personality style, Preserving, see chapter 3.

The mean values for the control group before and after the therapeutic intervention are as follow:

Table 4.23 Comparison of differences between the pre- and post-test mean scores of the control group on MIPS: Preserving

	N	Minimum	Maximum	Mean	Std. Deviation
Pre Preserv	17	32.0	100.0	58.588	26.3701
Post Preserv	17	13.0	100.0	52.882	29.4637

The differences between the pre- and post-test mean scores of the control group on MIPS: Preserving seem to be insignificant in terms of the criteria set out by Millon (1994). The pre-test mean scores (58.6) for the control al group match that of the category of significant prevalence of the personality style, Preserving. The post-test mean scores (52.9) for the control group match the category of significant prevalence of the personality style, Preserving (see Figure 4.12).

Figure 4.12 Comparison of differences between the pre- and post-test mean scores of the control group on MIPS: Preserving

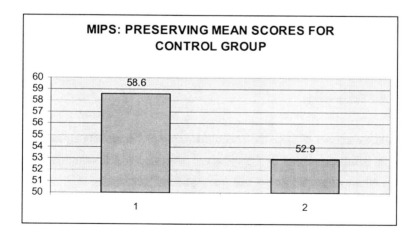

101

A Wilcoxon Signed Ranks Test which was used to determine the significance of difference between experimental variable on MIPS: Preserving before the intervention and after the intervention revealed that there is statistically not a significant difference between the pre-test scores and post-test scores of the control group (see table 4.24).

Table 4.24   Wilcoxon Signed Ranks Test for significance of differences between the pre- and post-test mean scores of the control group on MIPS: Preserving

		N	Mean Rank	Sum of Ranks	Post Preserv - Pre Preserv
Post Preserv - Pre Preserv	Negative Ranks	12	6.67	80.00	
	Positive Ranks	2	12.50	25.00	
	Ties	3			
	Total	17			Z= -1.727
	Asymp. Sig. (2-tailed)				.084

4.3.1.13 Significance of differences between the pre- and post- test mean scores of the experimental group on the personality style MIPS:Yielding

The prevalence scores (PS) on the Millon Inventory of Personality styles are regarded as being significant for PS values of 50 or higher. PS values that score lower than 50 are regarded as not being a significant personality style of the candidate. For a comprehensive description of the personality style, Yielding, see chapter 5.

The mean values for the experimental group before and after the therapeutic intervention are as follow:

Table 4.25   Comparison of differences between the pre- and post-test mean scores of the experimental group on MIPS: Yielding

	N	Minimum	Maximum	Mean	Std. Deviation
Pre Y	17	12.0	100.0	64.647	28.2819
Post Y	17	.0	100.0	49.941	28.0702

The differences between the pre- and post-test mean scores of the experimental group on MIPS: Yielding seem to be significant in terms of the criteria set out by Millon (1994). The pre-test mean scores (64.7) for the experiment al group match that of the category of significant prevalence of the personality style, Yielding. The post-test mean scores (49.9) for the experimental group match the category of insignificant prevalence of the personality style, Yielding (see Figure 4.13).

Figure 4.13 Comparison of differences between the pre- and post-test mean scores of the experimental group on MIPS: Yielding

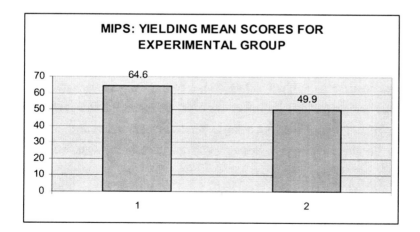

A Wilcoxon Signed Ranks Test which was used to determine the significance of difference between experimental variable on MIPS: Yielding before the intervention and after the intervention revealed that there is statistically not a significant difference between the pre-test scores and post-test scores of the experimental group (see table 4.26).

Table 4.26   Wilcoxon Signed Ranks Test for significance of differences between the pre- and post-test mean scores of the experimental group on MIPS: Yielding

		N	Mean Rank	Sum of Ranks	Post Y – Pre Y
Post Y - Pre Y	Negative Ranks	10	10.40	104.00	
	Positive Ranks	6	5.33	32.00	
	Ties	1			
	Total	17			Z= -1.862(a)
	Asymp. Sig. (2-tailed)				0.063

4.3.1.14 Significance of differences between the pre- and post- test mean scores of the control group on the personality style MIPS:Yielding

The prevalence scores (PS) on the Millon Inventory of Personality styles are regarded as being significant for PS values of 50 or higher. PS values that score lower than 50 are regarded as not being a significant personality style of the candidate. For a comprehensive description of the personality style, Yielding, see chapter 3.

The mean values for the control group before and after the therapeutic intervention are as follow:

Table 4.27 Comparison of differences between the pre- and post-test mean
scores of the control group on MIPS: Yielding

	N	Minimum	Maximum	Mean	Std. Deviation
Pre Y	17	31.0	100.0	62.824	26.0894
Post Y	17	17.0	100.0	56.882	26.1627

The differences between the pre- and post-test mean scores of the control group on MIPS: Yielding seem to be insignificant in terms of the criteria set out by Millon (1994). The pre-test mean scores (62.8) for the control group match that of the category of significant prevalence of the personality style, Yielding. The post-test mean scores (56.9) for the control group match the category of significant prevalence of the personality style, Yielding (see Figure 4.14).

Figure 4.14 Comparison of differences between the pre- and post-test mean
scores of the control group on MIPS: Yielding

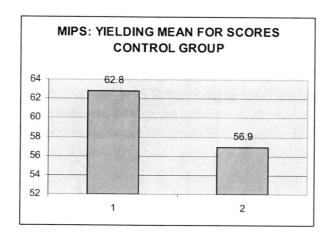

A Wilcoxon Signed Ranks Test which was used to determine the significance of difference between experimental variable on MIPS: Yielding before the intervention and after the intervention revealed that there is statistically not a significant difference between the pre-test scores and post-test scores of the control group (see table 4.28).

Table 4.28   Wilcoxon Signed Ranks Test for significance of differences between the pre- and post-test mean scores of the control group on MIPS: Yielding

		N	Mean Rank	Sum of Ranks	Post Y - Pre Y
Post Y- Pre Y	Negative Ranks	10	7.70	77.00	
	Positive Ranks	5	8.60	43.00	
	Ties	2			
	Total	17			Z= -.966
	Asymp. Sig. (2-tailed)				.334

4.3.1.15   Significance of differences between the pre- and post- test mean scores of the experimental group on the personality style MIPS:Complaining

The prevalence scores (PS) on the Millon Inventory of Personality styles are regarded as being significant for PS values of 50 or higher. PS values that score lower than 50 are regarded as not being a significant personality style of the candidate. For a comprehensive description of the personality style, Complaining, see chapter 3.

The mean values for the experimental group before and after the therapeutic intervention are as follow:

**Table 4.29 Comparison of differences between the pre- and post-test mean
scores of the experimental group on MIPS: Complaining**

	N	Minimum	Maximum	Mean	Std. Deviation
Pre Com	17	22.0	98.0	58.706	22.9504
Post Com	17	14.0	89.0	50.882	19.9214

The differences between the pre- and post-test mean scores of the experimental
group on MIPS: Complaining seem to be insignificant in terms of the criteria set out
by Millon (1994). The pre-test mean scores (58.7) for the experiment al group
match that of the category of significant prevalence of the personality style,
Complaining. The post-test mean scores (50.9) for the experimental group match
the category of significant prevalence of the personality style, Complaining (see
Figure 4.15).

**Figure 4.15 Comparison of differences between the pre- and post-test
mean scores of the experimental group on MIPS: Complaining**

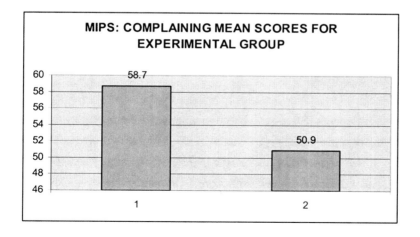

A Wilcoxon Signed Ranks Test which was used to determine the significance of difference between experimental variable on MIPS: Complaining before the intervention and after the intervention revealed that there is statistically not a significant difference between the pre-test scores and post-test scores of the experimental group (see table 4.30).

Table 4.30 Wilcoxon Signed Ranks Test for significance of differences between the pre- and post-test mean scores of the experimental group on MIPS: Complaining

		N	Mean Rank	Sum of Ranks	Post Com - Pre Com
Post Com - Pre Com	Negative Ranks	11	9.68	106.50	
	Positive Ranks	6	7.75	46.50	
	Ties	0			
	Total	17			Z= -1.421
	Asymp. Sig. (2-tailed)				.155

4.3.1.16 Significance of the differences between the pre- and post- test mean scores of the control group on the personality style MIPS:Complaining

The prevalence scores (PS) on the Millon Inventory of Personality styles are regarded as being significant for PS values of 50 or higher. PS values that score lower than 50 are regarded as not being a significant personality style of the candidate. For a comprehensive description of the personality style, Complaining, see chapter 3.

The mean values for the control group before and after the therapeutic intervention are as follow:

Table 4.31 Comparison of differences between the pre- and post-test mean scores of the control group on MIPS: Complaining

	N	Minimum	Maximum	Mean	Std. Deviation
Pre Com	17	20.0	100.0	68.235	26.5272
Post Com	17	16.0	100.0	66.118	24.4767

The differences between the pre- and post-test mean scores of the control group on MIPS: Complaining seem to be insignificant in terms of the criteria set out by Millon (1994). The pre-test mean scores (68.2) for the control group match that of the category of significant prevalence of the personality style, Yielding. The post-test mean scores (66.1) for the control group match the category of significant prevalence of the personality style, Yielding (see Figure 4.16).

Figure 4.16 Comparison of differences between the pre- and post-test mean scores of the control group on MIPS: Complaining

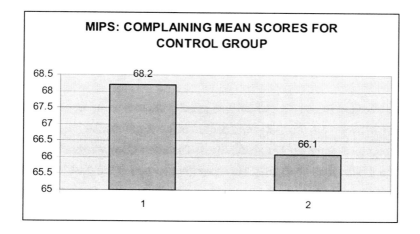

A Wilcoxon Signed Ranks Test which was used to determine the significance of difference between experimental variable on MIPS: Complaining before the intervention and after the intervention revealed that there is statistically not a significant difference between the pre-test scores and post-test scores of the control group (see table 4.32).

Table 4.32   Wilcoxon Signed Ranks Test for significance of differences between the pre- and post-test mean scores of the control group on MIPS: Complaining

		N	Mean Rank	Sum of Ranks	Post Com - Pre Com
Post Com - Pre Com	Negative Ranks	8	7.63	61.00	
	Positive Ranks	6	7.33	44.00	
	Ties	3			
	Total	17			Z= -.534
	Asymp. Sig. (2-tailed)				.594

4.3.1.17 Significance of differences between the pre- and post- test mean scores of the experimental group vs the control group on CFSQ- Secondary Traumatic Stress Disorder / Compassion Fatigue

A Wilcoxon Signed Ranks Test which was used to determine the significance of differences between the pre test mean scores of the experimental group vs. the control group on Secondary Traumatic Stress Disorder/ Compassion Fatigue show no significant difference (P=0.262). However the average of the post-test scores for the experimental group vs. the control group on Secondary Traumatic Stress Disorder/ Compassion Fatigue is significant (P=0.009).

Figure 4.17 Comparison of differences between the pre- and post-test mean scores of the experimental group vs. the control group on Secondary Traumatic Stress Disorder/ Compassion Fatigue

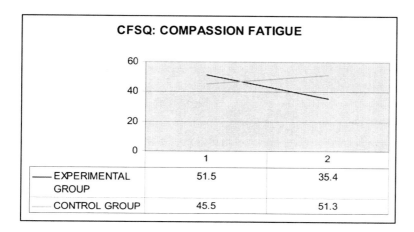

CFSQ: COMPASSION FATIGUE		
	1	2
EXPERIMENTAL GROUP	51.5	35.4
CONTROL GROUP	45.5	51.3

4.3.1.18 Significance of differences between the pre- and post- test mean scores of the experimental group vs the control group on CFSQ-Burnout

A Wilcoxon Signed Ranks Test which was used to determine the significance of differences between the pre test mean scores of the experimental group vs. the control group on CFSQ- Burnout show no significant difference (P=0.972). The average of the post-test scores for the experimental group vs. the control group on CSFQ-Burnout is significant (P=0.031).

Figure 4.18 Comparison of differences between the pre- and post-test mean scores of the experimental group vs. the control group on CFSQ: Burnout

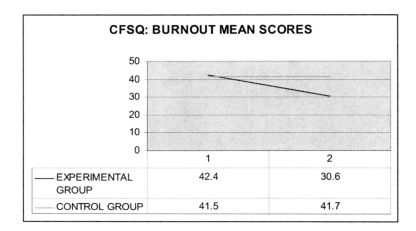

CFSQ: BURNOUT MEAN SCORES		
	1	2
—— EXPERIMENTAL GROUP	42.4	30.6
—— CONTROL GROUP	41.5	41.7

4.3.1.19 Significance of differences between the pre- and post- test mean scores of the experimental group vs the control group on CFSQ-Compassion Satisfaction

A Wilcoxon Signed Ranks Test which was used to determine the significance of differences between the pre test mean scores of the experimental group vs. the control group on CFSQ- Compassion Satisfaction show no significant difference (P=0.667). The average of the post-test scores for the experimental group vs. the control group on CFSQ- Compassion Satisfaction is not significant (P=0.986).

Figure 4.19 Comparison of differences between the pre- and post-test mean scores of the experimental group vs. the control group on CFSQ: Compassion Satisfaction

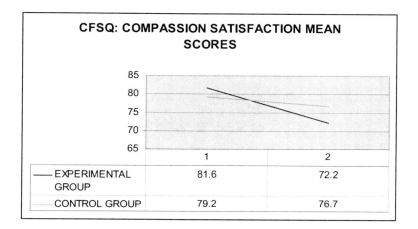

CFSQ: COMPASSION SATISFACTION MEAN SCORES

	1	2
—— EXPERIMENTAL GROUP	81.6	72.2
········· CONTROL GROUP	79.2	76.7

4.3.1.20 Significance of differences between the pre- and post- test mean scores of the experimental group vs the control group on LQ-Burnout

A Wilcoxon Signed Ranks Test which was used to determine the significance of differences between the pre test mean scores of the experimental group vs. the control group on LQ- Burnout show no significant difference (P=0.972). The average of the post-test scores for the experimental group vs. the control group on LQ- Burnout is not significant (P=0.148). Of interest is that (see figure 4.20) the post-test mean score of the experimental group fall into the category of modest risk vs. the post-test mean score of the control group falling into the category of significant risk.

Figure 4.20 Comparison of differences between the pre- and post-test mean scores
of the experimental group vs. the control group on LQ- Burnout

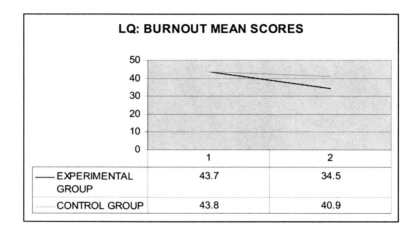

4.3.1.21 Significance of differences between the pre- and post- test mean
scores of the experimental group vs the control group on
MIPS:Enhancing

A Wilcoxon Signed Ranks Test which was used to determine the significance of differences between the pre test mean scores of the experimental group vs. the control group on MIPS: Enhancing show no significant difference (P=0.469). The average of the post-test scores for the experimental group vs. the control group on MIPS: Enhancing is not significant (P=0.704).

What is of interest (see figure 4.20) is that the experimental group mean scores improved from non-significance (PS=43.2) to a post-test mean score of significance prevalence (PS= 51.9). The control group mean scores remained insignificant both pre-test (PS=42.1) as well as post-test (PS= 46.5).

Figure 4.21 Comparison of differences between the pre- and post-test mean scores of the experimental group vs. the control group on MIPS: Enhancing

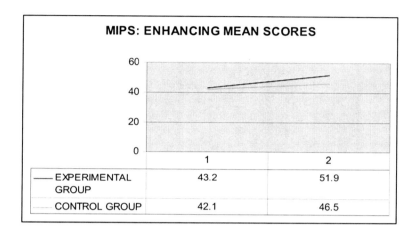

MIPS: ENHANCING MEAN SCORES	1	2
EXPERIMENTAL GROUP	43.2	51.9
CONTROL GROUP	42.1	46.5

4.3.1.22 Significance of differences between the pre- and post- test mean scores of the experimental group vs the control group on MIPS:Preserving

A Wilcoxon Signed Ranks Test which was used to determine the significance of differences between the pre test mean scores of the experimental group vs. the control group on MIPS: Preserving show no significant difference (P=1.00). The average of the post-test scores for the experimental group vs. the control group on MIPS: Preserving is not significant (P=0.877).

What is of interest (see figure 4.22) is that the experimental group mean scores decreased from significance (PS=53.7) to a post-test mean score of non-significant prevalence (PS= 44.7). The control group mean scores remained significant both pre-test (PS=58.6) as well as post-test (PS= 52.9).

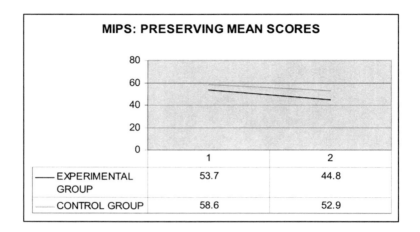

MIPS: PRESERVING MEAN SCORES

	1	2
—— EXPERIMENTAL GROUP	53.7	44.8
········· CONTROL GROUP	58.6	52.9

4.3.1.23 Significance of differences between the pre- and post- test mean scores of the experimental group vs the control group on MIPS:Yielding

A Wilcoxon Signed Ranks Test which was used to determine the significance of differences between the pre test mean scores of the experimental group vs. the control group on MIPS: Yielding show no significant difference (P=0.704). The average of the post-test scores for the experimental group vs. the control group on MIPS: Yielding is non-significant (P=0.468).

What is of interest (see figure 4.23) is that the experimental group mean scores decreased from significance (PS=64.6) to a post-test mean score of non-significant prevalence (PS= 49.9). The control group mean scores remained significant both pre-test (PS=62.8) as well as post-test (PS= 56.9).

116

Figure 4.23 Comparison of differences between the pre- and post-test mean scores of the experimental group vs. the control group on MIPS: Yielding

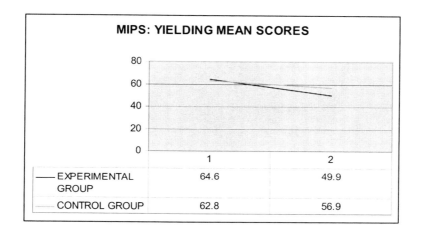

MIPS: YIELDING MEAN SCORES

	1	2
EXPERIMENTAL GROUP	64.6	49.9
CONTROL GROUP	62.8	56.9

4.3.1.24 Significance of differences between the pre- and post- test mean scores of the experimental group vs the control group on MIPS:Complaining

A Wilcoxon Signed Ranks Test which was used to determine the significance of differences between the pre test mean scores of the experimental group vs. the control group on MIPS: Complaining show no significant difference (P=0.248). The average of the post-test scores for the experimental group vs. the control group on MIPS: Complaining is not significant (P=0.060).

What is of interest (see figure 4.24) is that the experimental group mean scores decreased from significance (PS=58.7) to a post-test mean score of marginal significant prevalence (PS= 50.9). The control group mean scores remained significant both pre-test (PS=68.2) as well as post-test (PS= 66.1).

117

Figure 4.24 **Comparison of differences between the pre- and post-test mean scores
of the experimental group vs. the control group on MIPS: Complaining**

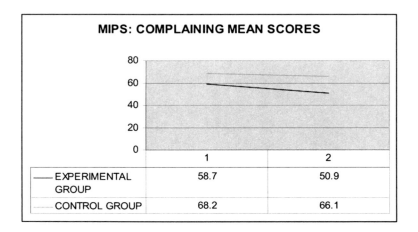

MIPS: COMPLAINING MEAN SCORES		
	1	2
—— EXPERIMENTAL GROUP	58.7	50.9
·········· CONTROL GROUP	68.2	66.1

4.4 Concluding remarks

This chapter reviewed the results of the pre-test and post-test results both intra-
group as well as inter-group. The following chapter discusses the results in detail in
terms of the objectives of this research. This chapter laid out the results of the
various tests. No attempt was made in this chapter to interpret the results. The
following and final chapter, Chapter Five, discusses the results as well as the
merits and the limitations of the study and recommendations for future studies are
made.

CHAPTER FIVE

DISCUSSION

5.1 Introduction

Secondary traumatic stress disorder has become a significant phenomenon in the South African context of emergency rescue workers. Numerous studies regarding the incidence of secondary traumatic stress disorder have been published (see chapter 2). It can be concluded from the research literature (Figley, 2003) so far that emergency rescue workers who are exposed to chronic critical incidents are at significant risk of contracting secondary traumatic stress disorder. Although not all rescue workers contract this condition after exposure to a traumatic event, those who do present with it seem to need some kind of intervention.

No spontaneous improvement has been cited in the literature as seems to be the case with some incidents of an acute stress disorders (Bisson, 2003), thus implying the need for therapeutic interventions in diagnosed cases.

Fewer studies on the treatment of secondary traumatic stress disorder exist (see chapter two). Yet a review of the literature on the treatment of secondary traumatic stress disorder in the South African context with quantitive statistical results on its efficacy yielded no results.

Of the intervention programs that are on offer the common themes that are apparent are: subjective experiences, cognitive perceptions and coping behaviours that act as primary, secondary and tertiary interventions. The most comprehensive program was designed by Gentry et al (2003), namely the Accelerated Recovery

Program (ARP)/Pathways aftercare model. Although the model seems to be comprehensive, no statistical data is supplied to underscore its efficacy, nor are individual needs and competencies regarded in its implementation.

The single session intervention programmes (Mitchell, 1983; Dyregov, 1989; Raphael, 1986), as discussed in the literature review, that have become popular in the treatment of work trauma and general acute stress disorders have no proven benefit to persons that presents with secondary traumatic stress disorders.

Although the multiple stressor debriefing model (Armstrong et al, 1991) supports individual; approaches vs. group interventions, no specific attention to individual needs and attributes is proposed. Still the general stages of treatment are followed, without any data to substantiate self-proclaimed benefit.

The Constructivist Self Developmental Theory treatment program developed by Saakvitne and Pearlman (1992) propose an extensive self-care treatment program for rescue workers that present with more chronic secondary traumatic stress disorder or vicarious traumatization. Although extensive mention is made of individual interventions, no mention is made of personality assessment to customize solution plans.

The closest reference to explaining individual differences in the prevalence of STSD and it's recovery process can be found in Valent's (2003) theory of survival strategies (see chapter two). Again no reference is made to specific personality traits that would possibly be derived from such an approach.

Marmar et al (1996) did extensive research on the role that personality traits play in PTSD etiology and recovery. However no mention in the literature can be found regarding personality styles that contribute to the origin of neither STSD nor its treatment.

The objective of this study was to evaluate the effectiveness of an Action Centered Personological Treatment Plan; that encompasses cognitive behavioural principles, on the treatment of Secondary Traumatic Stress Disorder (STSD)/compassion fatigue as well as Burnout among South African emergency rescue workers.

Through exposure of the experimental group to the Action Centered Personological Treatment Plan, the desired objective was a decrease in the symptoms of STSD/compassion fatigue. The treatment program also aimed at treating the co-morbid symptom of emotional and physical exhaustion found with burnout without reducing the prevalence of compassion satisfaction.

In broad terms the hypotheses of this study were robustly supported by the statistical data. The principle hypothesis was supported by the data, as the experimental group showed a decrease in STSD/compassion fatigue variables and co-morbid symptoms of burnout following the intervention program of three sessions and a trial period of six weeks, without significantly reducing their sense of compassion satisfaction. Similar decreases were not detected in the control group. Instead marginal increases in scores on STSD were found with the control group.

For the purpose of this study, the following hypotheses were generated and tested:

1. An Action Centred Personological Treatment Program will significantly reduce symptoms of secondary traumatic stress disorder/ compassion fatigue, in the experimental group from pre- to post-testing, as well as show significantly fewer symptoms than the control group at post-testing.

2. An Action Centred Personological Treatment Program will significantly reduce symptoms of burnout, in the experimental group from pre- to post-testing, as well as show significantly fewer symptoms than the control group at post-testing.

121

3. An Action Centred Personological Treatment Program will not significantly affect the condition of compassion satisfaction in a negative way, in the experimental group from pre- to post-testing, as well as score significantly higher than the control group at post-testing.

An analysis of the data shows that the changes expected to occur, based on the theoretical prediction of the impact of the Action Centred Personological Treatment Program (as described in chapter three), did in fact occur regarding hypotheses one and two. In order to test the above hypotheses 34 subjects were tested for STSD/compassion fatigue, the co-morbid symptom of burnout and compassion satisfaction. The group was randomly signed to an experimental group and control group.

Subjects who were assigned to the experimental group (17 members) were exposed to the individual treatment programme of three sessions over a six week period. The control group (17 members) received no treatment for six weeks. After the six week period both groups were given a three month "breather" period. After the three month period both groups were re-tested.

5.2 The efficacy of an action centered personological treatment program for STSD/Compassion Fatigue in terms of specific components and compassion satisfaction

5.2.1 CSFQ- Secondary Traumatic Stress Disorder/ Compassion Fatigue

Secondary Traumatic Stress Disorder/ Compassion Fatigue results from exposure to critical incidents in the attempt to rescue trauma victims. Reduction of this condition results, among others, in a decrease in generalized fear, intrusive thoughts, flashbacks, avoidance behaviour, persistent arousal both emotionally and somatically, changes regarding beliefs and attitudes about their own abilities and the world, and other work related trauma symptoms.

The hypothesis regarding the efficacy of the Action Centred Personological Treatment Program for STSD/ compassion fatigue was supported in the sense that there was a significant improvement by means of a significant decrease in the CFSQ-scores for STSD/ compassion fatigue symptomatology for the experimental group, both in terms of intra-group and inters group scores.

In order to prove that the intervention did in fact decrease symptoms of STSD/compassion fatigue, it was necessary to prove that the experimental and control groups were the same at the beginning of the experimental design. The results revealed that there was no significant difference between the experimental group and control group on the prevalence of STSD/compassion fatigue as both scored in the category of extreme high risk of STSD/compassion fatigue.

The experimental group showed a significant sustained improvement in a reduction of STSD/compassion fatigue symptoms after a three month period following the intervention program of three sessions. Scores reduced from the category of extreme high risk to the category of moderate risk of STSD/compassion fatigue.

These scores were also significantly better than that of the control group. The control group did not score significantly better between the pre-and post test scores. Both scores were in the category of extreme high risk of STSD/compassion fatigue. This provides support for the hypothesis that without intervention there is no improvement expected in the symptoms of STSD/compassion fatigue.

5.2.2 Burnout

Burnout occurs in response to chronic high occupational stress in conjunction with poor life skills. It can result in feelings of hopelessness and de-motivation in dealing with work demands. Onset is gradual and results from a sense that one's efforts make no difference. Two test-scores were used in the study to determine the significance of this condition. They are the CFSQ-score, as well as the British Columbia Life Style Questionnaire (LQ).

i)   CFSQ-Burnout

The results showed that there was no significant difference between the experimental group and control group scores at the onset of the study. Both groups' scores on the CFSQ scale for burnout registered in the category of moderate risk of burnout. Accordingly the groups were found to be the same at the beginning of the study.

The statistical analysis revealed that there was a significant difference between the experimental group before the intervention and the experimental group three months after the intervention. The scores changed from the category of moderate stress to the category of extremely low risk of burnout. These findings provide support for the hypothesis that the Action Centered Personological Treatment Program will lead to a significant reduction of burnout symptoms.

Although the experimental group and the control groups scored the same at the beginning of the study there was no significant difference between the CFSQ scores for burnout for the control group before the intervention and the control group three months after the intervention. This provides support for the hypothesis that symptoms of burnout do not improve spontaneously without any intervention.

There was a significant difference between the experimental group versus the control group scores on CFSQ-burnout three months after the intervention. This further contributes to strengthen the hypothesis that symptoms of burnout improve more significantly after being exposed to an Action Centered Personological Treatment Program than without.

ii) LQ-Burnout

Both the experimental group and the control group scores on the LQ- scale for burnout registered in the category of significant risk of burnout. Accordingly the groups were found to be the same at the beginning of the study.

The statistical analysis revealed that there was a significant difference between the experiment al group before the intervention and the experiment al group three months after the intervention. The scores changed from the category of significant stress to the category of modest risk of burnout. These findings provide support for the hypothesis that the Action Centered Personological Treatment Program will lead to a significant reduction of burnout symptoms.

The experimental group and the control groups scored the same at the beginning of the study. Statically there was no significant difference between the control group before the intervention and the control group three months after the intervention. This provides support for the hypothesis that symptoms of burnout do not improve spontaneously without any intervention.

Statically there was no significant difference between the experimental group and the control group scores on LQ-burnout three months after the intervention. However there was a qualitative difference in the scores as the experimental groups LQ-scores dropped significantly from a category of significant risk of burnout to a category of modest risk of burnout, while the control group scores remained relatively unchanged. This further contributes to strengthen the hypothesis that symptoms of burnout improve after being exposed to an Action Centered Personological Treatment Program than without. The lack of statistical significance in comparison to the CFSQ-burnout values may question the sensitivity or lack of it of the LQ-questionnaire

5.2.3 CFSQ-Compassion Satisfaction

Compassion satisfaction refers to the rescue workers' ability to maintain a belief system that what they are doing helps other people in ways that can even be liberating. This, according to Stamm (2003) can add to the individual's resilience and act as a protective barrier against possible STSD/ Compassion fatigue. This would imply that there would be an inverse relation between compassion satisfaction and STSD/ compassion fatigue.

In order to prove that the intervention did in fact decrease symptoms of compassion satisfaction, it was necessary to prove that the experimental and control groups were the same at the beginning of the experimental design. The results revealed that there was no significant difference between the experimental group and control group on the prevalence of compassion satisfaction as both score in the category of modest potential for compassion satisfaction.

The experimental group showed no significant reduction in their potential for compassion satisfaction after a three month period following the intervention program of three sessions. Scores remained in the category of modest potential for compassion satisfaction.

These scores were also no better than that of the control group. The control group did not score significantly different between the pre-and post test scores. Both scores were in the category of modest potential for compassion satisfaction.

This provides partial support for the hypothesis regarding the efficacy of the Action Centred Personological Treatment Program for compassion satisfaction in the sense that there was no significant change in the CFSQ-scores for Compassion Satisfaction for the experimental group before and after the intervention.

What is of interest is that both the experimental group and the control group scored statistically on par before and after the intervention. This contradicts the hypothesis that an experimental group who had been exposed to an Action Centred Personological Treatment Plan will score significantly higher in their potential for compassion satisfaction than the control group who had received no intervention.

It also challenges Stamm's (2003) claim that the construct compassion satisfaction aids in containing and/or preventing the escalation of STSD/compassion fatigue, as in this case it practically played no part in preventing or aggravating STSD/co passion fatigue. According to the research results obtained it seems that compassion satisfaction plays no role in protecting rescue workers from STSD/compassion fatigue. Furthermore it seems that the Action Centred Personological Treatment Plan does not improve one's potential for compassion satisfaction.

An alternative proposition could be that due to the chronic psycho-social stresses that were mentioned in chapter three regarding poor management and negative corporate culture then construct, compassion satisfaction, was under constant duress. The construct was therefore possibly unable to assist the individuals to remain resilient while being exposed to these constant stresses which were beyond their perceived control.

However the intervention program was able to make a difference which again begs the legitimacy of this construct.

5.2.4 Millon Inventory of Personality Styles (MIPS)

The prevalence scores (PS) on the Millon Inventory of Personality Styles are regarded as being significant for PS values of 50 or higher. PS values that score lower than 50 are regarded as not being a significant personality style of the candidate.

Although none of the twenty four personality styles of the MIPS scored statistically significantly different before and after the intervention program for both the experimental group and control group, there were some qualitative differences in the intra-group scores for the experimental group.

i) Enhancing

The personality style, Enhancing, refers to one's attitudes and behaviours designed to foster and enrich life, generate joy, pleasure, contentment, and fulfilment; thereby strengthening one's capacity to remain competent physically and mentally. Persons who posses this personality style are often driven by the desire to enrich their lives and seek invigorating experiences and challenges, all to magnify their vitality and viability.

On the personality style, Enhancing, the PS values for the experimental group improved from the category of non-significance (PS=43) to the category of significant prevalence (PS=52).

This personality style is similar to the construct of resilience which forms part of compassion satisfaction as proposed by Stamm (2003). Although her construct showed no difference in prevalence before and after the intervention, Millon's (1994) personality style of Enhancing did on a qualitative basis.

ii) Preserving

The personality style, Preserving, refers to a tendency to focus one's attention on potential threats to one's emotional and physical security, an expectation of and heightened alertness to the signs of potential negative feedback that can lead one to disengage from everyday relationships and pleasurable experiences. Although individuals who posses this personality style may be successful at avoiding unnecessary risks and danger, it comes at a price of narrowing your range of positive emotions and joyful experiences.

On the personality style, Preserving, the PS values for the experimental group improved from the category of significance (PS=54) to the category of non-significant prevalence (PS=43).

This personality style is similar to the construct of STSD/compassion fatigue as proposed by Sabin-Farrell and Turpin (2003). Both their construct (quantitively on the CFSQ values) and Millon's (1994) personality style of Preserving (qualitively) showed a significant improvement before and after the intervention program.

iii) Yielding

The personality style, Yielding, refers to a disposition to act in a subservient and self-abasing manner. Placing oneself in an inferior light or abject position, one may act unassertive, if not servile. One's behavior may render ineffective the efforts of others to assist one and causes one to bypass opportunities for rewards and to fail repeatedly to achieve, despite possessing abilities to do so.

On the personality style, Yielding, the PS values for the experimental group improved from the category of significance (PS=65) to the category of non-significant prevalence (PS=49.9).

129

This construct is often seen as the opposite of assertiveness and resilience. Accordingly, its qualitive change may provide support for the hypothesis that resilience can be seen as a protective measure in managing STSD/compassion satisfaction.

The results as obtained by the MIPS scores suggest that there is some correlation, if not statistically significant, between the scores for STSD/compassion fatigue, burnout, compassion satisfaction and the former personality styles. Because of the low statistical correlation it is proposed that the MIPS values are best suited for diagnostic and treatment purposes, rather than for pre- and post-testing the efficacy of the Action Centered Personological Treatment Program.

5.3 The cost-effectiveness of an action centered personological treatment program

The theoretical basis that forms the paradigm of the intervention program is discussed in chapter two. The various theoretical approaches and intervention techniques presented, help understand how a personological treatment program incorporating the principles of cognitive behavioural therapy would help to reduce the prevalence of STSD/ compassion fatigue as well as co-morbid symptoms of burnout. In this study it was found that there were significant decreases in the prevalence of STSD/compassion fatigue and in the co-morbid symptoms of burnout.

A great deal of emphasis is placed on individual personality styles regarding the assessment of specific cognitive behavioural needs that the individual may posses. This would then aid in the formulation of specific cognitive behavioural techniques suited to the individual's personality styles and abilities to treat the former needs with regard to STSD/compassion fatigue and burnout, including, controlled breathing, emotive/irrational thought stopping, guided-self dialogue and cognitive restructuring (specifically regarding self beliefs/life scripts).

Specific treatment programs were designed to help the individuals improve their creative problem solving potential, thus enhancing their emotional resilience and self-confidence. As their locus of control (self-confidence) improves it would contribute to immunize them against future secondary trauma symptoms.

One of the main aims of this research was to develop an Action Centered Personological Treatment Program that would treat the symptoms of STSD/compassion fatigue related to critical incidents. The goal of the intervention was to decrease the prevalence of STSD/compassion fatigue symptoms in both the shortest amount of time as well as ensure that the changes that are realized remain consistent over time. This was a distinctive challenge as emergency rescue workers in South Africa work under constant threat of being exposed to critical incidents while being under huge financial constraints.

According to Valent (2003) the continuous exposure to critical incidents is not enough to cause the manifestation of PTSD/compassion fatigue symptoms. Thus a treatment program needed to be designed in order to attend to this unique problem. The treatment program focused on employing clinical personology and cognitive behavioural therapy to treat the individual needs and causes of symptoms of STSD/compassion fatigue (see chapter four) in response to critical incidents.

The Action Centered Personological Treatment Program was found to be effective on a post-test level with regard to the central variable STSD/compassion fatigue as well as the co-morbid variable of burnout. The results of the treatment program were significantly positive. There was a substantial decrease on the variables of both STSD/compassion fatigue and burnout after exposure to the therapeutic intervention.

The control group remained the same between the pre-test and the post-test. This is contrary to the findings of Ehlers, Mayou and Bryant (1998) and Bisson (2003) that many symptoms of acute and chronic PTSD will remit in time. The conflict in results in these findings may be related to the fact that the emergency rescue workers are continuously exposed to the risk of STSD/compassion fatigue through their occupational hazards of critical incidents. The stress levels are further aggravated by perceived poor working conditions and ineffective management practices.

Drawing on the theory of Figley (1983) STSD/compassion fatigue is distinguished from other anxiety disorders by a critical incident in the occupational lives of emergency rescue workers. This leads to an emotional duress experienced by individuals having close contact with a trauma survivor, especially concerned family members, it is viewed as a natural response to a survivor's traumatic material with which emergency staff may identify or empathise (Figley & Kleber, 1995). The symptoms are viewed as being similar to that of PTSD (see table 1.1).

Controlled breathing and emotive/irrational thought stopping exercises are used in order to break the intrusive imagery of the critical incidents as well as the avoidance symptoms. According to Foa and Meadows (1997) systematic desensitization has been found to be successful in the treatment of fear and anxiety.

Guided self dialogue and cognitive restructuring techniques have been employed in disputing negative perceptions about subjects' self concept, others and the world. This combined with creative potential development and personalised stress management skills training contributed to a general increase in emotional resilience and self-confidence.

Compared to the numerous studies mentioned in chapter two, what made this intervention unique is that individual personality styles (from MIPS) were used to identify subjective needs and accordingly personalise solution plans. The principle that was followed through-out was on being able to take action. By being empowered with specific skills on what to do this made it easier for participants to identify with the solution plans and take greater ownership for their part in this recovery process.

By giving the subjects both verbal and written feedback on their personality functioning in regard to STSD/compassion fatigue and then customizing cognitive behavioural plans to attend to their specific personological needs, it is possible to convey much more therapeutic information in a short time span, without sacrificing on lost information. The subjects as it were trained to manage their own symptoms on a continuous basis.

Although the study focused on specific personality style needs and abilities, it cannot segregate each technique and relate it specifically to the reduction of a specific STSD/compassion fatigue symptom, the results provide strong support that the Action Centred Personological Treatment Program was successful in treating STSD/compassion fatigue and co-morbid symptoms of burn-out related to emergency rescue workers.

The effects were evident three months after the intervention program were completed and the subjects had been exposed to further critical incidents, i.e. the effects of the treatment program were evident over the medium term for all variables.

The treatment programme consisted of three therapeutic sessions over a six week period, which is regarded as short-term therapy. The former provides support for the cost-effectiveness of the Action Centred Personological Treatment Program in the treatment of STSD/compassion fatigue in emergency rescue workers. It would seem that this treatment program is indeed highly effective and can be easily used by professionals.

5.4 Limitations to this study

Some of the limitations of this study are focused around methodical issues. Due to the demands that were put on the subjects regarding shifts and training it were only possible to have three sessions with each subject of the experimental group. Had there been opportunity for three more sessions further improvement in symptomatology would have been expected.

It could not be conclusively proven through the results of this study that a personological centred cognitive behavioural program is the most effective treatment of STSD/compassion fatigue for emergency rescue workers. The study merely provides the first exploratory quantitive data that a personological cognitive behavioural program is an effective treatment for STSD/compassion fatigue.

What could not be confirmed through the results of this study was the effectiveness of specific techniques on specific STSD/compassion fatigue symptoms. It is therefore difficult to isolate and measure for the effectiveness of certain personological centred cognitive behavioural techniques on specific symptoms of STSD/compassion fatigue for emergency rescue workers. Further research in this field is required.

5.5 Recommendations

Recommendations for future research would include, narrowing down the focus of techniques used in the program, in order to measure and identify more specifically what techniques target which symptoms of STSD/compassion fatigue.

Future research in the area of STSD/compassion fatigue among emergency rescue workers in South Africa could investigate the effectiveness of personological centred cognitive behavioural therapy in the treatment of PTSD and multiple PTSD, among for example police officers and soldiers.

Comparisons between the Action Centred Personological Treatment Program and other treatment models should be encouraged to conclusively determine the effectiveness of each treatment modality in the treatment of STSD/compassion fatigue.

Further research into the management of STSD/compassion fatigue on a managerial level is indicated. The assessment and recruitment of staff in South Africa does not include any risk assessment o for STSD/compassion fatigue. Future studies in this matter and subsequent pre-morbid life skills training would be welcome.

REFERENCES

American Psychiatric Association. (1980). Diagnostic and statistical manual of mental disorders (Third edition). Washington, DC: Author.

American Psychiatric Association. (1994). Diagnostic and statistical manual of mental disorders (Fourth edition). Washington, DC: Author.

Armstrong, K., O'Callahan, W. & Marmar, C.R. (1991). Debriefing Red Cross disaster personnel: the multiple stressor debriefing model. Journal of Traumatic Stress, 4: 581-593.

Bisson, J.I. (2003). Single-session early psychological interventions following traumatic events. Clinical Psychology Review, 23(3): 481-499.

Bisson, J.I., Jenkins, P.L., Alexander, J. & Bannister, C. (1997). Randomised trial of psychological debriefing for victims of acute burn trauma. British Journal of Psychiatry, 171:78-81.

Bower, G. (1981). Mood and memory. American Psychologist, 36: 129-148.

Brewin, C.R., Andrews, B. & Valentine, J.D. (2000). Meta-analysis of risk factors for posttraumatic stress disorder in trauma-exposed adults. Journal of Consulting and Clinical Psychology, 68 (5): 748-766.

Brewin, C.R., Dalgleish,T. & Joseph, S. (1996). A dual representation theory of posttraumatic stress disorder. Psychological Review, 103 (4): 670-686.

Bryant, R.A., Harvey, A.G., Dang, S.T., Sackville, T. and Basten, C. (1998). Treatment of acute stress disorder: a comparison of cognitive-behavioural therapy and supportive counselling. Journal of Consulting and Clinical Psychology, 66: 862-866.

Burns, R.N. & Harm, N.J. (1993). Research: Emergency nurses' perceptions of critical incidents and stress debriefing. Journal of emergency nursing,19(5): 431-436.

Clark, L.A., Watson, D. & Mineka, S. (1994). Temperament, personality and the mood and anxiety disorders. Journal of Abnormal Psychology, 103: 103-116.

Clark, G.M. & Cooke, D. (2004). A basic course in statistics (Fifth edition). London: Arnold.

Clayton, P.J. & Darvish, H.S. (1979). Course of depressive symptoms following the stress of bereavement. In Barret, J. (Ed.) Stress and Mental Disorder. New York: Raven Press.

Clohessey, S. & Ehlers, A. (1999). PTSD symptoms, response to intrusive memories and coping in ambulance service workers. British Journal of Clinical Psychology, 38: 251-265.

Dalgleish, T. (1999). Cognitive theories of posttraumatic stress disorder. In W.Yule (Ed.) Post-traumatic stress disorders. Concepts and therapy. Chichester: John Wiley & Sons.

Department of Health, 1998. Our healthier nation: a contract of health. Stationary Office: London

De Silva, P. (1999). Cultural aspects of posttraumatic stress disorder. In W.Yule (Ed.) Post-traumatic stress disorders. Concepts and therapy. Chichester: John Wiley & Sons.

De Silva, P. & Marks, M. (1999). Intrusive thinking in posttraumatic stress disorder. In W.Yule (Ed.) Post-traumatic stress disorders. Concepts and therapy. Chichester: John Wiley & Sons.

Donner, L. & Schonfield, J. 1975). Affect contagion in beginning psychotherapists. Journal of Clinical Psychology, 31: 332-339.

Durham, T.W., McCammon, S.L. & Jackson Alison, E. (1985). The psychological impact of disaster on rescue personnel. Annals of Emergency Medicine 14 (7): 664-668.

Dyregrov, A. (1989). Caring for helpers in disaster situations: psychological debriefing. Disaster Management, 2: 2-30.

Dyregrov, A. (1998). Psychological debriefing- an effective method? Traumatology, 4: p.2 (Article 1)

Ehlers, A. & Clark, D.M. (2000). A cognitive model of posttraumatic stress disorder. Behaviour Research and Therapy, 38 (4): 319-345.

Ehlers, A., Mayou, R.A. & Bryant, B. (1998). Psychological predictors of chronic posttraumatic stress disorder after motor vehicle accidents. Journal of Abnormal Psychology, 107 (3): 508-519.

Ehlers, A. & Steil, R. (1995). Maintenance of intrusive memories in PTSD: a cognitive approach. Behavioural and Cognitive Psychotherapy, 23: 217-249.

Figley, C.R. (1983). Catastrophes: An overview of family reactions. In C.R. Figley & M.cCubbin (Eds.) Stress and the family: vol.2. Coping with catastrophe (pp3-10). New York: Brunner/Mazel.

Figley, C.R. (1995). Systematic traumatization: Secondary traumatic stress disorder: An overview. In C.R. Figley (Ed.). Compassion fatigue: coping with secondary traumatic stress disorder in those who treat the traumatized (pp1-20). New York Brunner/Maazel.

Figley, C.R. & Kleber, R.J. (1995). Beyond the "victim": Secondary traumatic stress. In R.J. Kleber, C.R. Figley & B.P.R. Gersons (Eds.), Beyond trauma: Cultural and societal dynamics (pp75-98). New York: Plenum.

Figley,C.R.& Stamm, B.H. (1996). Psychometric review of the Compassion Fatigue Self Test. In B.H. Stamm (Ed.), Measurement of stress, trauma, and adaptation. Lutherville: Sidran Press.

Figley, C.R. (2003). Introduction. In C.R. Figley (Ed.) Treating compassion fatigue. New York: Brunner-Routledge.

Foa, E.B. & Meadows, E.A. (1997). Psychological Treatments For Posttraumatic Stress Disorder: A Critical Review. Annual Review of Psychology, 48: 449-480.

Frolkey, C.A. (1992, May/June). Critical incidents and traumatic events; the differences. EAP Digest, 12(4).

Gentry, J.E., Baranowsky, A.B. & Dunning, K. (2003). ARP: The accelerated recovery program (ARP) for compassion fatigue. In C.R. Figley (Ed.) Treating compassion fatigue. New York: Brunner-Routledge.

Green, B.L., Grace, M.C., Lindy, J.D., Gleser, G.C. & Leonard, B.A. (1990). Risk factors for PTSD in a general sample of Vietnam veterans. American Journal of Psychiatry, 147(6): 729-733.

Grevin, F. (1996). Postraumatic stress disorder, ego defence mechanisms, and empathy among urban paramedics. Psychological Reports, 79: 483-495.

Hagh-Shenas, H., Goldstein, L. & Yule, W. (1999). Psychobiology of posttraumatic stress disorder. In W.Yule (Ed.) Post-traumatic stress disorders. Concepts and therapy. Chichester: John Wiley & Sons.

Hatfield, E., Cacioppo, J.T. & Rapson, R.L. (1994.) Emotional contagion. Studies in emotion and social interaction. Paris: Cambridge University Press.

Helzer, J.E., Robins, L.N. & Wish, E. 1979). Depression in Vietnam veterans and civilian controls. American Journal of Psychiatry, 136: 526-529.

Hesse, A.R. (2002). Secondary trauma: How working with trauma survivors affects therapists. Clinical Social Work Journal, 30(3): 1-17.

Hodgkinson, P.E. & Stewart, M. (1998). Coping with catastrophe. A handbook of post-disaster psychosocial aftercare. Second edition. London: Routledge.

Horowitz, M.J. (1986.) Stress response syndromes. Second edition. London: Jason Aronson Inc.

Horowitz, M.J. & Wilner, N. (1981). Life events, stress and coping. In Poon, L. (Ed.) Aging in the 80's. Washington D.C.: American Psychological Association.

Jackson, S.E., Schwab, R,L. & Schuler, R.S. 1986. Toward an understanding of the burnout phenomenon. Journal of Applied Psychology, 71: 630-640.

Janoff-Bulman, R. (1985). The aftermath of victimization: Rebuilding shattered assumptions. In C.R. Figley (Ed.) <u>Trauma and its wake</u>. New York: Brunner/Mazel.

Jenkins, S.R. & Baird, S. (2002). Secondary traumatic stress and vicarious traumatization: A validational study. <u>Journal of Traumatic Stress, 15(5)</u>: 423-432.

Kaplan, H.I. & Sadock, B.J. (1998). <u>Kaplan and Sadock's synopsis of psychiatry: behavioural sciences, clinical psychiatry-eighth edition</u>. Maryland: Williams @ Wilkins.

Labovitz, S. & Hagedorn, R. (1981). <u>Introduction to Social Research: Third edition.</u> New York: McGraw- Hill Book Co.

Laposa, J.M. & Alden, L.E. (2001). Posttraumatic stress disorder in the emergency room: exploration of a cognitive model. <u>Behaviour Research and Therapy, uncorrected proof.</u>

Lazarus, R.S. & Folkman, S. (1984). <u>Stress, Appraisal, and Coping.</u> New York: Springer.

Mahoney, M.J. (1981). Psychotherapy and human change processes. In Harvey J.H. & Parks, M.M. (Eds.) <u>Psychotherapy Research and Behaviour Change, Master lecture series</u>. Washington D.C.: American Psychological Association.

Marmar, C.R.; Weiss, D.S.; Metzler, M.A. & Delucchi, K. (1996). Characteristics of emergency services personnel related to peritraumatic dissociation during critical incident exposure. <u>American Journal of Psychiatry, 153(7)</u>: 94-110.

Maslach, C. (1982). <u>Burnout: The cost of caring</u>. Englewood Cliffs, New Jersey: Prentince-Hall.

Maslach, C. (1987). Burnout research in the social services: A critique. In D.F. Gillespie (Ed.). Burnout among social workers (pp95-105). New York: Haworth Press.

McCammon, S., Durham, T.W., Jackson Alison, E. & Williamson, J.E. (1987). Emergency workers' cognitive appraisal and coping with traumatic events. Journal of Traumatic Stress, 1(3): 353-372.

McCann, I.L. & Pearlman, L.A. (1990). Vicarious traumatization: a framework for understanding the psychological effects of working with victims. Journal of Traumatic Stress, 3(1): 131-149.

McCann, I.L., Sakheim, D.K. & Abrahamson, D.J. (1988). Trauma and victimization: A model of psychological adaptation. The Counselling Psychologist, 16 (4): 531-594.

McFarlane A.C. (1989). The aetiology of posttraumatic morbidity: predisposing, precipitation and perpetuating factors. British Journal of Psychiatry, 154: 221-228.

Miller, K.I., Stiff, J.B. & Ellis, B.H. (1998). Communication and empathy as precursors to burnout among human service workers. Communication Monographs, 55: 250-265.

Millon, T. (1994). Millon Index of Personality Styles. Manual. San Antonio: Harcourt Brace & Co.

Mitchell, J.T. (1983). When disaster strikes…the critical incident debriefing process. Journal of Emergency Medical Services, 8: 36-39.

Mitchell, J.T. (1988). Effects of stress management training on paramedic coping styles and perceived stress levels. Dissertation Abstracts International, 45(5): 1617-B.

Mitchell, J.T. & Everly, G.S. (1995). Critical incident stress debriefing: an operations manual for the prevention of traumatic stress among emergency services and disaster workers. Maryland: Chevron Publishing.

Moos, R.H. & Billings, A.G. (1982). Conceptualizing and measuring coping resources and processes. In Goldberg, L. & Breznitz, S. (Eds.) Handbook of Stress: Theoretical and Clinical Aspects. New York: The Free Press.

Moos, R.H. & Schaefer, J.A. (1986). overview and perspective. In R.H. Moos (Ed.) Coping with Life Crises. New York: Plenum.

Moran, C. & Britton, N.R. (1994). Emergency work experience and reactions to traumatic incidents. Journal of Traumatic Stress, 7(4): 575-585.

Myers, D & Wee, D.F. (2003). Strategies for managing mental health worker stress. In C.R. Figley (Ed.) Treating compassion fatigue. New York: Brunner-Routledge.

National Institute of Mental Health (2002). Mental health and mass violence: evidence-based early psychological intervention for victims/survivors of mass violence. A workshop to reach consensus on best practices. NIH Publication no 02-5138. Washington: U.S. Printing Office.

Neuman, D.A. & Gamble, S.J. (1995). Issues in the professional development of psychotherapists: counter transference and vicarious traumatization in the new trauma therapist. Psychotherapy, 32: 341-347.

Oppenheim, A.N. (1992). Questionnaire Design, Interviewing and Attitude Measurement: New Edition. London: Pinter Publishers.

Paivio, A. (1986). Mental Representations: A Dual Coding Approach. New York: Oxford University Press.

Pearlman, P.L. & MacCann, P.S. (1995). Vicarious traumatization: an empirical study of the effects of trauma work on trauma therapists. Professional psychology: Research and Practice, 26(6): 558-565.

Pearlman, L.A. & Saakvitne, K.W. (1995). Trauma and the Therapist: Countertransference and Vicarious Traumatization in Psychotherapy with Incest Survivors. New York: W.W. Norton & Co.

Piaget, J. (1971). Psychology and Epistemology: Toward a Theory of Knowledge. New York: Viking.

Raphael, B. (1986). When disaster strikes: a handbook for caring professionals. London: Hutchenson.

Rose, S.,Bisson, J. & Wessley, S. 2002. Psychological debriefing for prevention of post traumatic stress disorder (PTSD) (Cochrane review). In The Cochrane Library, Issue2, 2002. Update Software: Oxford.

Saakvitne, K.W. & Pearlman, L.A. (1992). Transforming the Pain: A Workbook on Vicarious Traumatization. New York: W.W. Norton & Co.

Sabin-Farrell, R.& Turpin, G. (2003). Vicarious traumatization: implications for the mental health of health workers? Clinical Psychology Review, 23(3): 449-480.

Schauben, L.J. & Frazier, P.A. (1995). Vicarious traumatzation: The effects on female counsellors of working with sexual violence survivors. Psychology of Woman Quarterly, 19: 49-64.

144

Schnurr, P.P.; Friedman, M.J. & Rosenberg, S.D. (1993). Preliminary MMPI scores as predictors of combat related PTSD symptoms. American Journal of Psychiatry, 150 (3): 479-483.

Shalev, A.Y., Bonne, O. & Eth, S. (1996). Treatment of Posttraumatic Stress Disorder: A Review. Psychosomatic Medicine, 58: 165-182.

Spatz, C. (1993). Basic Statistics: Tales of Distributions. Fifth Edition. Pacific Grove: Brooks/Cole Publishing Co.

Stamm, B.H. (2003). Measuring compassion satisfaction as well as fatigue: Developmental history of the compassion satisfaction and fatigue test. In C.R. Figley (Ed.) Treating compassion fatigue. New York: Brunner-Routledge.

Sawyer, C.M. (2001). A survey of team members who participate in traumatic event group psychological debriefings. Dissertations Abstracts International: Section B: The Sciences and Engineering; Jun 2001; 61 (11-B): 6148.

Summerfield, D. (2001). The invention of post-traumatic stress disorder and the social usefulness of a psychiatric category. British Medical Journal, 322: 95-98.

Taylor, S.E. (1983). Adjustment to threatening events: A theory of cognitive adaptation. American Psychologist, 38(11): 1161-1173.

Thrasher,S. & Dalgleish, T. (1999). The use of information processing paradigms to investigate posttraumatic stress disorder: A review of the evidence. In W.Yule (Ed.) Post-traumatic stress disorders. Concepts and therapy. Chichester: John Wiley & Sons.

Thompson, J. & Suzuki,I. (1991). Stress in ambulance workers. Disaster management, 3: 193-197.

Trippany, R.L., White Kress, V.E. & Allan Wilcoxon, S. (2004). Preventing Vicarious Trauma: What counsellors should know when working with trauma survivors. Journal of Counselling and Development, 82(1): 1-15.

Valent, P. (2003). Diagnosis and treatment of helper stresses, traumas, and illnesses. In C.R. Figley (Ed.) Treating compassion fatigue. New York: Brunner-Routledge.

Van Minnen, A. & Keijsers, G.P.J. (2000). A controlled study into the (cognitive) effects of exposure treatment on trauma therapists. Journal of Behaviour and Experimental Psychiatry, 31(3-4): 189-200.

Wagner, D., Heinrichs, M. & Ehlert, U. (1998). Prevalence of symptoms of posttraumatic stress disorder in German professional fire-fighters. American Journal Of Psychiatry, 155(12): 1727-1732.

Weiss, D.S., Marmar, C.R., Metzler, T.J. & Ronfeldt, H.M. (1995). Predicting symptomatic distress in emergency services personnel. Journal of Consulting and Clinical Psychology, 63(3): 361-368.

Wheeler, H.H. (1998). Nurse occupational stress research 5: sources of determinants of stress. British Journal of Nursing, 7(1): 40-43.

Williams, R.(1999). Personality and posttraumatic stress disorder. In W.Yule (Ed.) Post-traumatic stress disorders. Concepts and therapy. Chichester: John Wiley & Sons.

Williams, R., Hodgkinson, P., Joseph, S. & Yule, W. (1995). Attitudes to emotion, crisis support and distress 30 months after the capsize of a passenger berry. Crisis intervention, 1: 209-214.

Williams, R.& Joseph, S. (1999). Conclusions; An integrative psychosocial model of PTSD. In W.Yule (Ed.) Post-traumatic stress disorders. Concepts and therapy. Chichester: John Wiley & Sons.

Wilson, J.P, Harel, Z. & Kahana, B. (1988). Human adaptation to extreme stress. From the Holocaust to Vietnam. New York: Plenum Press.

Wolpe, J. (1958). Psychotherapy by reciprocal inhibition. Stanford: Stanford University Press.

Woodall, S.J. (1999). Ask not why the wounded fall, but how the valiant continue to march: New theory on work-related stress management in the fire service. Dissertation Abstracts international Section A: Humanities & Social Sciences; Mar 1999; 59(9-A): 3665.

Yehuda, R. & McFarlane, A.C. (1995). Conflict between current knowledge about posttraumatic stress disorder and its original conceptual basis. American Journal of Psychiatry,152(12): 1705-1713.

Zellars, K.L., Perrewé, P.L. & Hochwarter, W.A. (2000). Burnout in health care: The role of the five factors of personality. Journal of Applied Social Psychology, 30 (8): 1570-1598.

ADDENDUM 1

Descriptive Statistics of Experimental Group

	N	Minimum	Maximum	Mean	Std. Deviation
Gender	17	1.0	1.0	1.000	.0000
Age	17	25.0	39.0	31.529	4.3749
Ethnicity	17	1.0	4.0	2.000	1.1726
Marital	17	1.0	3.0	1.353	.7019
Position	17	1.0	3.0	1.706	.5879
Experience	17	1.0	14.0	5.647	3.9677
Academic	17	1.0	4.0	2.882	.6002
Pre LQ Burnout	17	31.0	71.0	43.706	10.0919
Post LQ Burnout	17	15.0	52.0	34.529	12.4153
Pre CFSQ Compassion Fatigue	17	29.0	74.0	51.529	14.2921
Post CFSQ Compassion Fatigue	17	8.0	56.0	35.353	12.3235
Pre CFSQ Burnout	17	19.0	55.0	42.353	8.9229
Post CFSQ Burnout	17	8.0	49.0	30.647	11.4069
Pre CFSQ Compassion Satisfaction	17	56.0	117.0	81.588	16.6022
Post CFSQ Compassion Satisfaction	17	6.0	119.0	72.235	29.1709
Pre MIPS Enhancing	17	1.0	70.0	43.176	18.9118
Post MIPS Enhancing	17	13.0	86.0	51.882	23.0540
Pre MIPS Preserving	17	22.0	100.0	53.706	22.0391
Post MIPS Preserving	17	9.0	95.0	44.765	22.4096
Pre MIPS Modifying	17	.0	83.0	61.706	19.5505
Post MIPS Modifying	17	15.0	87.0	58.294	22.6571
Pre MIPS Accommodating	17	26.0	100.0	48.471	17.4145

Post MIPS Accommodating	17	9.0	87.0	46.529	21.0033
Pre MIPS Individuating	17	.0	100.0	68.882	28.0844
Post MIPS Individuating	17	15.0	100.0	61.412	20.8088
Pre MIPS Nurturing	17	11.0	93.0	57.824	23.9667
Post MIPS Nurturing	17	.0	87.0	43.412	27.3566
Pre MIPS Extraversing	17	9.0	89.0	48.059	21.0964
Post MIPS Extraversing	17	6.0	80.0	40.353	21.0652
Pre MIPS Introversing	17	9.0	93.0	55.824	22.1394
Post MIPS Introversing	17	20.0	85.0	52.412	17.5002
Pre MIPS Sensing	17	3.0	100.0	62.706	26.5277
Post MIPS Sensing	17	5.0	89.0	64.941	20.8371
Pre MIPS Intuiting	17	15.0	92.0	42.176	21.2522
Post MIPS Intuiting	17	5.0	94.0	39.294	22.9013
Pre MIPS Thinking	17	8.0	100.0	64.765	24.4528
Post MIPS Thinking	17	38.0	100.0	68.824	19.4719
Pre MIPS Feeling	17	15.0	85.0	48.647	21.2542
Post MIPS Feeling	17	.0	89.0	42.765	19.7849
Pre MIPS Systematizing	17	9.0	80.0	47.294	25.2853
Post MIPS Systematizing	17	9.0	80.0	54.000	23.7855
Pre MIPS Innovating	17	9.0	67.0	39.765	15.7144
Post MIPS Innovating	17	1.0	84.0	35.471	20.3474
Pre MIPS Retiring	17	36.0	100.0	58.647	19.0982
Post MIPS Retiring	17	9.0	100.0	62.000	23.7144
Pre MIPS Outgoing	17	9.0	83.0	48.647	23.3772
Post MIPS Outgoing	17	16.0	78.0	48.824	16.0087
Pre MIPS Hesitating	17	36.0	100.0	65.000	24.0520
Post MIPS Hesitating	17	20.0	87.0	49.706	17.0102
Pre MIPS Asserting	17	11.0	79.0	49.000	20.5609
Post MIPS Asserting	17	23.0	83.0	58.059	16.9354
Pre MIPS Dissenting	17	24.0	98.0	61.235	21.7616
Post MIPS Dissenting	17	26.0	89.0	51.294	18.6406

Pre MIPS Conforming	17	37.0	100.0	64.000	17.3961
Post MIPS Conforming	17	6.0	89.0	57.941	22.8814
Pre MIPS Yielding	17	12.0	100.0	64.647	28.2819
Post MIPS Yielding	17	.0	100.0	49.941	28.0702
Pre MIPS Controlling	17	7.0	100.0	54.235	29.6153
Post MIPS Controlling	17	13.0	100.0	60.000	23.6485
Pre MIPS Complaining	17	22.0	98.0	58.706	22.9504
Post MIPS Complaining	17	14.0	89.0	50.882	19.9214
Pre MIPS Agreeing	17	.0	100.0	52.824	26.9194
Post MIPS Agreeing	17	.0	92.0	52.765	26.4233
Pre MIPS Positive Impression	17	.0	9.0	2.941	2.5610
Post MIPS Positive Impression	17	.0	8.0	3.412	2.1231
Pre MIPS Negative Impression	17	2.0	8.0	4.765	1.6781
Post MIPS Negative Impression	17	2.0	7.0	4.000	1.3693
Post LQ Burnout	17	1.00	4.00	2.4118	1.06412
LQ Burnout	17	2.00	5.00	3.0000	.79057
Compassion Fatigue	17	2.00	5.00	4.4706	.87447
Post Compassion Fatigue	17	1.00	5.00	3.2941	1.64942
Burn Out	17	1.00	5.00	4.1765	1.13111
Post Burn Out	17	1.00	5.00	2.8235	1.55062
Compassion Satisfaction	17	1.00	4.00	2.5294	1.00733
Post Compassion Satisfaction	17	1.00	5.00	2.3529	1.22174
Valid N (listwise)	17				

ADDENDUM 2

Descriptive Statistics for Control Group

	N	Minimum	Maximum	Mean	Std. Deviation
Gender	17	1.0	2.0	1.118	.3321
Age	17	24.0	51.0	32.647	6.7448
Ethnicity	17	1.0	4.0	1.765	.8314
Marital	17	1.0	3.0	1.588	.9393
Position	17	1.0	5.0	2.118	1.2187
Experience	17	2.0	16.0	7.118	4.1965
Academic	17	2.0	4.0	3.059	.6587
Pre LQ Burnout	17	19.0	70.0	43.824	12.7193
Post LQ Burnout	17	17.0	68.0	40.882	12.8932
Pre CFSQ Compassion Fatigue	17	6.0	85.0	45.471	17.0518
Post CFSQ Compassion Fatigue	17	9.0	85.0	51.294	19.6366
Pre CFSQ Burnout	17	7.0	68.0	41.471	17.1505
Post CFSQ Burnout	17	7.0	83.0	41.706	17.8142
Pre CFSQ Compassion Satisfaction	17	48.0	123.0	79.176	19.6604
Post CFSQ Compassion Satisfaction	17	29.0	111.0	76.706	23.2426
Pre MIPS Enhancing	17	.0	80.0	42.059	28.6192
Post MIPS Enhancing	17	.0	86.0	46.471	30.0835
Pre MIPS Preserving	17	32.0	100.0	58.588	26.3701
Post MIPS Preserving	17	13.0	100.0	52.882	29.4637
Pre MIPS Modifying	17	.0	89.0	58.647	29.8893
Post MIPS Modifying	17	.0	84.0	47.941	33.5996
Pre MIPS Accommodating	17	13.0	100.0	51.000	24.7790

Post MIPS Accommodating	17	21.0	100.0	55.059	26.6657
Pre MIPS Individuating	17	15.0	100.0	76.529	27.0419
Post MIPS Individuating	17	15.0	100.0	72.471	25.7661
Pre MIPS Nurturing	17	8.0	89.0	48.765	22.7473
Post MIPS Nurturing	17	.0	89.0	43.412	25.1248
Pre MIPS Extraversing	17	.0	83.0	45.471	25.3479
Post MIPS Extraversing	17	.0	80.0	38.882	28.4975
Pre MIPS Introversing	17	23.0	97.0	61.647	24.3514
Post MIPS Introversing	17	20.0	100.0	63.353	27.7893
Pre MIPS Sensing	17	14.0	89.0	61.882	21.1302
Post MIPS Sensing	17	9.0	94.0	62.412	24.9451
Pre MIPS Intuiting	17	12.0	100.0	53.353	24.5712
Post MIPS Intuiting	17	12.0	81.0	46.471	21.3457
Pre MIPS Thinking	17	12.0	100.0	72.824	28.8514
Post MIPS Thinking	17	12.0	100.0	73.471	26.6742
Pre MIPS Feeling	17	4.0	92.0	47.588	21.1100
Post MIPS Feeling	17	.0	89.0	43.176	25.9163
Pre MIPS Systematizing	17	.0	87.0	54.765	31.1659
Post MIPS Systematizing	17	.0	92.0	48.176	29.8061
Pre MIPS Innovating	17	3.0	77.0	44.059	23.5464
Post MIPS Innovating	17	.0	87.0	40.706	22.3684
Pre MIPS Retiring	17	14.0	100.0	61.824	26.2041
Post MIPS Retiring	17	28.0	100.0	70.706	26.2459
Pre MIPS Outgoing	17	.0	93.0	55.471	30.8851
Post MIPS Outgoing	17	.0	87.0	43.647	36.9644
Pre MIPS Hesitating	17	22.0	100.0	60.882	28.9285
Post MIPS Hesitating	17	20.0	100.0	56.706	30.7180
Pre MIPS Asserting	17	.0	100.0	58.294	27.5131
Post MIPS Asserting	17	.0	87.0	49.059	29.7961
Pre MIPS Dissenting	17	15.0	100.0	71.176	24.8174
Post MIPS Dissenting	17	18.0	100.0	68.412	27.6067

Pre MIPS Conforming	17	12.0	92.0	64.412	28.3572
Post MIPS Conforming	17	1.0	91.0	55.588	29.0109
Pre MIPS Yielding	17	31.0	100.0	62.824	26.0894
Post MIPS Yielding	17	17.0	100.0	56.882	26.1627
Pre MIPS Controlling	17	25.0	100.0	67.412	22.3916
Post MIPS Controlling	17	9.0	100.0	65.118	26.5233
Pre MIPS Complaining	17	20.0	100.0	68.235	26.5272
Post MIPS Complaining	17	16.0	100.0	66.118	24.4767
Pre MIPS Agreeing	17	.0	95.0	48.706	23.5286
Post MIPS Agreeing	17	.0	95.0	47.118	25.9757
Pre MIPS Positive Impression	17	.0	9.0	4.059	3.0917
Post MIPS Positive Impression	17	.0	8.0	3.882	2.5220
Pre MIPS Negative Impression	17	1.0	9.0	5.471	2.1828
Post MIPS Negative Impression	17	1.0	9.0	4.529	2.7184
Post LQ Burnout	17	1.00	5.00	2.8235	1.07444
LQ Burnout	17	1.00	5.00	3.0588	1.02899
Compassion Fatigue	17	1.00	5.00	4.4118	1.12132
Post Compassion Fatigue	17	1.00	5.00	4.2941	1.15999
Burn Out	17	1.00	5.00	3.7647	1.75105
Post Burn Out	17	1.00	5.00	3.8824	1.61564
Compassion Satisfaction	17	1.00	5.00	2.4118	1.22774
Post Compassion Satisfaction	17	1.00	4.00	2.4706	1.00733
Valid N (listwise)	17				

Lightning Source UK Ltd.
Milton Keynes UK
09 July 2010

156790UK00007B/10/P